CHALLENGES AND SUCCESSES IN REDUCING HEALTH DISPARITIES

Workshop Summary

Jennifer A. Cohen, *Rapporteur*

Roundtable on Health Disparities

Board on Population Health and Public Health Practice

INSTITUTE OF MEDICINE
OF THE NATIONAL ACADEMIES

THE NATIONAL ACADEMIES PRESS
Washington, D.C.
www.nap.edu

THE NATIONAL ACADEMIES PRESS 500 Fifth Street, N.W. Washington, DC 20001

NOTICE: The project that is the subject of this report was approved by the Governing Board of the National Research Council, whose members are drawn from the councils of the National Academy of Sciences, the National Academy of Engineering, and the Institute of Medicine.

This study was supported by multiple contracts and grants between the National Academy of Sciences and the Agency for Healthcare Research and Quality and the Office of Minority Health, U.S. Department of Health and Human Service (Contract HHSP23320042509XI, TO#11); California Endowment (Contract 20052634); California HealthCare Foundation (Contract 06-1213); Commonwealth Fund (Contract 20060048); Connecticut Health Foundation (unnumbered grant); Ford Foundation (Contract 1050-0152,FF5H003); Healthcare Georgia Foundation (unnumbered grant); The Henry J. Kaiser Family Foundation (Contract 01-1149-810); Kaiser Permanente (Contract 20072164); Merck (unnumbered grant); Missouri Foundation for Health (Contract 06-0022-HPC); Robert Wood Johnson Foundation (Contract 56387); and W. K. Kellogg Foundation (Contract P0123822). Any opinions, findings, conclusions, or recommendations expressed in this publication are those of the author(s) and do not necessarily reflect the view of the organizations or agencies that provided support for this project.

International Standard Book Number-13: 978-0-309-11690-9
International Standard Book Number-10: 0-309-11690-2

Additional copies of this report are available from the National Academies Press, 500 Fifth Street, N.W., Lockbox 285, Washington, DC 20055; (800) 624-6242 or (202) 334-3313 (in the Washington metropolitan area); Internet, http://www.nap.edu.

For more information about the Institute of Medicine, visit the IOM home page at: **www.iom.edu.**

Printed in the United States of America

The serpent has been a symbol of long life, healing, and knowledge among almost all cultures and religions since the beginning of recorded history. The serpent adopted as a logotype by the Institute of Medicine is a relief carving from ancient Greece, now held by the Staatliche Museen in Berlin.

Suggested citation: IOM (Institute of Medicine). 2008. *Challenges and successes in reducing health disparities: Workshop summary.* Washington, DC: The National Academies Press.

"Knowing is not enough; we must apply.
Willing is not enough; we must do."
—Goethe

INSTITUTE OF MEDICINE
OF THE NATIONAL ACADEMIES

Advising the Nation. Improving Health.

THE NATIONAL ACADEMIES

Advisers to the Nation on Science, Engineering, and Medicine

The **National Academy of Sciences** is a private, nonprofit, self-perpetuating society of distinguished scholars engaged in scientific and engineering research, dedicated to the furtherance of science and technology and to their use for the general welfare. Upon the authority of the charter granted to it by the Congress in 1863, the Academy has a mandate that requires it to advise the federal government on scientific and technical matters. Dr. Ralph J. Cicerone is president of the National Academy of Sciences.

The **National Academy of Engineering** was established in 1964, under the charter of the National Academy of Sciences, as a parallel organization of outstanding engineers. It is autonomous in its administration and in the selection of its members, sharing with the National Academy of Sciences the responsibility for advising the federal government. The National Academy of Engineering also sponsors engineering programs aimed at meeting national needs, encourages education and research, and recognizes the superior achievements of engineers. Dr. Charles M. Vest is president of the National Academy of Engineering.

The **Institute of Medicine** was established in 1970 by the National Academy of Sciences to secure the services of eminent members of appropriate professions in the examination of policy matters pertaining to the health of the public. The Institute acts under the responsibility given to the National Academy of Sciences by its congressional charter to be an adviser to the federal government and, upon its own initiative, to identify issues of medical care, research, and education. Dr. Harvey V. Fineberg is president of the Institute of Medicine.

The **National Research Council** was organized by the National Academy of Sciences in 1916 to associate the broad community of science and technology with the Academy's purposes of furthering knowledge and advising the federal government. Functioning in accordance with general policies determined by the Academy, the Council has become the principal operating agency of both the National Academy of Sciences and the National Academy of Engineering in providing services to the government, the public, and the scientific and engineering communities. The Council is administered jointly by both Academies and the Institute of Medicine. Dr. Ralph J. Cicerone and Dr. Charles M. Vest are chair and vice chair, respectively, of the National Research Council.

www.national-academies.org

ROUNDTABLE ON HEALTH DISPARITIES*

---

*IOM forums and roundtables do not issue, review, or approve individual documents. The responsibility for the published workshop summary rests with the workshop rapporteur and the institution.

Jeffrey Levi, Executive Director, Trust for America's Health, Washington, DC

James C. Lewin, Chief Executive Officer, American College of Cardiology, Washington, DC

Jane Isaacs Lowe, Senior Program Officer, Robert Wood Johnson Foundation, Princeton, NJ

Richard K. Murray, Vice President, External Medical and Scientific Affairs, U.S. Human Health, Merck and Company, Inc., North Wales, PA

Gary D. Nelson, President, Healthcare Georgia Foundation, Atlanta, GA

Samuel Nussbaum, Executive Vice President and Chief Medical Officer, WellPoint, Inc., Indianapolis, IN

Michael W. Painter, Senior Program Officer, Robert Wood Johnson Foundation, Princeton, NJ

David P. Pryor, Medical Director, Aetna; Founder, Black Women Health.com, Thousand Oaks, CA

Steve M. Pu, General Surgeon, Missouri Foundation for Health, Kennett, MO

Kyu Rhee, Director, Office of Innovation and Program Coordination, National Center on Minority Health and Health Disparities, National Institutes of Health, Bethesda, MD

Mark D. Smith, President and CEO, California Health Care Foundation, Oakland

Mildred Thompson, Senior Director, PolicyLink, Center for Health and Place, Oakland, CA

Pattie Tucker, Lead Health Scientist, Community and Health Program, National Center for Chronic Disease Prevention and Health Promotion, Centers for Disease Control and Prevention, Atlanta, GA

Winston F. Wong, Medical Director, Community Benefit Director, Disparities Improvement and Quality Initiatives, Kaiser Permanente Federation, Oakland, CA

Terri D. Wright, Program Director, Health Policy, W. K. Kellogg Foundation, Battle Creek, MI

IOM Board on Population Health and Public Health Practice Liaisons

Samuel So, Professor, Stanford School of Medicine, Stanford University, Stanford, CA

William A. Vega, Professor, Department of Family Medicine, David Geffen School of Medicine, University of California, Los Angeles

Staff

Faith Mitchell, Senior Program Officer (through July 2007)
Jennifer A. Cohen, Program Officer (July 2007 through the present)
Rose Marie Martinez, Board Director
Thelma L. Cox, Senior Program Assistant
Christie Bell, Financial Officer
Christine McShane, Editor
Hope Hare, Administrative Assistant

Reviewers

This report has been reviewed in draft form by individuals chosen for their diverse perspectives and technical expertise, in accordance with procedures approved by the National Research Council's Report Review Committee. The purpose of this independent review is to provide candid and critical comments that will assist the institution in making its published report as sound as possible and to ensure that the report meets institutional standards for objectivity, evidence, and responsiveness to the study charge. The review comments and draft manuscript remain confidential to protect the integrity of the deliberative process. We wish to thank the following individuals for their review of this report:

Sharon E. Barrett, Association of Clinicians for the Underserved
Anne C. Beal, The Commonwealth Fund
Howard K. Koh, Harvard School of Public Health
Brian D. Smedley, Opportunity Agenda

Although the reviewers listed above have provided many constructive comments and suggestions, they were not asked to endorse the final draft of the report before its release. The review of this report was overseen by **Dr. Melvin Worth.** Appointed by the Institute of Medicine, he was responsible for making certain that an independent examination of this report was carried out in accordance with institutional procedures and that all review comments were carefully considered. Responsibility for the final content of this report rests entirely with the author and the institution.

Contents

Preface

In early 2007, the Institute of Medicine of the National Academies convened the Roundtable on Health Disparities to increase the visibility of racial and ethnic health disparities as a national problem, further the development of programs and strategies to reduce disparities, foster the emergence of leadership on this issue, and track promising activities and developments in health care that could lead to dramatically reducing or eliminating disparities. The Roundtable on Health Disparities includes representatives from the health professions, state and local government, foundations, philanthropy, academia, advocacy groups, and community-based organizations. Its mission is to facilitate communication across sectors and—above all—to generate action. Through national and local activities, the Roundtable strives to advance the goal of eliminating health disparities.

On July 31, 2007, the first workshop of the Roundtable on Health Disparities was held at Harris-Stowe State University in St. Louis, Missouri. To help stimulate new thinking about solutions and to inform its future meetings and discussions, the Roundtable brought together a diverse group of participants from a variety of fields to discuss racial and ethnic differences in life expectancy in the United States. Measured in terms of life expectancy, tens of millions of Americans experience levels of health that are more typical of middle- and low-income developing countries. These mortality differences are caused primarily by chronic diseases and injuries with well-established risk factors and are potentially amenable to intervention. The goals of the workshop were to increase the Roundtable's understanding of (1) the importance of differences in life expectancy within the United States,

(2) the reasons for the differences, and (3) the implications of this information for programs and policy makers.

This workshop provided the Roundtable members and sponsors with an opportunity to hear from a diverse group of people from across the country and to engage in an open dialogue about relevant issues and concerns related to reducing health disparities. Workshop participants offered different points of view and shared unique approaches for reducing disparities. While some of the workshop participants work on reducing disparities in health care, others strive to alleviate health disparities by addressing factors that determine a person's overall health, called the social or nonmedical determinants of health. This workshop provided an open forum during which representatives from these two disparate groups could share their evidence, research, experiences, and knowledge and, together with other workshop attendees, strategize actionable goals, remedies, and solutions for reducing health disparities.

ACKNOWLEDGMENTS

The Roundtable on Health Disparities would like to thank all of the workshop participants for their individual contributions to this workshop. The participants' willingness to share their time and expertise helped to inform the attendees and led to frank discussions about disparities in the United States. We would like to thank Drs. Horowitz and Lawlor for collaborating on a background paper that was commissioned by the Roundtable for this workshop. Their paper, "Community Approaches to Addressing Health Disparities," is in Appendix D. We would also like to thank Dr. Murray for providing the Roundtable with a copy of his paper "Eight Americas: Investigating Disparities Across Races, Counties, and Race-Counties in the United States" to further clarify the material in his presentation. Dr. Murray's published paper is in Appendix C. Presenters' biosketches and a listing of workshop participants can be found in Appendix B.

We would also like to extend our appreciation to Dr. Henry Givens, President of Harris-Stowe State University, for hosting the workshop in the Bank of America Theater at Emerson Performance Center on the Harris-Stowe State University Campus. We are also indebted to Dr. James Kimmey, President and Chief Executive Officer of the Missouri Foundation for Health, for sponsoring this workshop and for Dr. Kimmey's tireless efforts to ensure that the workshop was a success. Special thanks are also extended to Damon Green from the Missouri Foundation for Health for all of his hard work and exceptional organizational skills.

The Roundtable on Health Disparities would also like to thank IOM staff for their ongoing efforts to support the work of the Roundtable.

Sincere gratitude is extended to Dr. Rose Marie Martinez, the Director of the Board on Population Health and Public Health Practice; Dr. Faith Mitchell, for coordinating and overseeing the formation of the Roundtable and for planning and organizing this workshop; Jennifer Cohen, for her dedication to writing this workshop summary and for her oversight and management of the Roundtable after Faith's departure; and Thelma Cox, for skillfully overseeing all of the administrative responsibilities. We would also like to acknowledge the work of IOM staff members Christie Bell, Lara Andersen, Tia Carter, and Hope Hare for their ongoing assistance and support. We also gratefully acknowledge the efforts of IOM Anniversary Fellow, Roderick King, for reviewing early drafts of this summary and providing helpful advice.

Finally, we would like to thank all the sponsors who make the Roundtable on Health Disparities a reality. Financial support for this Roundtable was provided by the Agency for Healthcare Research and Quality and the Office of Minority Health, U.S. Department of Health and Human Services; the California Endowment; the California HealthCare Foundation; the Commonwealth Fund; the Connecticut Health Foundation; the Ford Foundation; the Healthcare Georgia Foundation; the Henry J. Kaiser Family Foundation; Kaiser Permanente; Merck; the Missouri Foundation for Health; the Robert Wood Johnson Foundation; and the W. K. Kellogg Foundation.

Dr. Nicole Lurie, *Chair*
Roundtable on Health Disparities

List of Acronyms

BRFSS	Behavioral Risk Factor Surveillance System
CBP	community-based planning
CBPR	community-based participatory research
CDC	Centers for Disease Control and Prevention
CEO	chief executive officer
CHW	community health worker
CLAS	cultural and linguistically appropriate services
CTSA	Clinical Translational Science Award
GAVI	Global Alliance for Vaccines and Immunization
HRSA	Health Resources and Services Administration
LISC	Local Initiatives Support Corporation
MTO	Move to Opportunity
NCHS	National Center for Health Statistics
NHANES	National Health and Nutrition Examination Survey
NIH	National Institutes of Health
REACH	Racial and Ethnic Approaches to Community Health
YRBS	Youth Risk Behavior Survey

1

Introduction[1]

In early 2007, the Institute of Medicine (IOM) of the National Academies convened the Roundtable on Health Disparities to increase the visibility of racial and ethnic health disparities as a national problem, further the development of programs and strategies to reduce disparities, foster the emergence of leadership on this issue, and track promising activities and developments in minority care that could lead to dramatically reducing or eliminating disparities. The Roundtable on Health Disparities includes representatives from the health professions, state and local government, foundations, philanthropy, academia, advocacy groups, and community-based organizations. Its mission is to facilitate communication across sectors and—above all—to generate action. Through national and local activities, the Roundtable strives to advance the goal of eliminating health disparities.

The Roundtable focuses on the disparities experienced by African Americans, Hispanics, Native Americans, Alaska Natives, Asians, and Pacific Islanders. These disparities are reflected in the frequency with which these groups experience such diseases as cancer, AIDS and HIV infection, cardiovascular disease, infant mortality, asthma, stroke, and diabetes. They are also reflected in difficulties experienced in accessing health care services, as well as in differences in health outcomes. Altogether, these disparities result in shorter life expectancy and reduced quality of life. If not tackled effec-

[1] The planning committee's role was limited to planning the workshop, and the workshop summary has been prepared by the workshop rapporteur as a factual summary of what occurred at the workshop.

tively now, health disparities could result in even more preventable deaths and disability as the racial and ethnic diversity of the country grows.

Through its convening capacity and by holding public workshops at different locations across the nation, the Roundtable on Health Disparities aspires to advance understanding of health disparities and explore solutions for ending them. In doing so, it endeavors to make a lasting contribution to the quality of life for some of this country's most vulnerable groups.

ABOUT THE WORKSHOP

On July 31, 2007, the first workshop of the Roundtable on Health Disparities was held at the Bank of America Theater at Emerson Performance Center on the campus of Harris-Stowe State University in St. Louis, Missouri. To help stimulate new thinking about solutions and to inform its future meetings and discussions, the Roundtable brought together a diverse group of participants from a variety of fields to discuss racial and ethnic differences in life expectancy in the United States. Measured in terms of life expectancy, tens of millions of Americans experience levels of health that are more typical of middle- and low-income developing countries. These mortality differences are caused primarily by chronic diseases and injuries with well-established risk factors and are potentially amenable to intervention. The goals of the workshop were to increase the Roundtable's understanding of (1) the importance of differences in life expectancy within the United States, (2) the reasons for the differences, and (3) the implications of this information for programs and policy makers.

To specifically address the issues pertaining to U.S. life-expectancy rates, the Roundtable invited Dr. Christopher Murray, director of the Institute for Health Metrics and Evaluation at the University of Washington, to discuss his recent paper, "Eight Americas: Investigating Mortality Disparities Across Races, Counties, and Race-Counties in the United States" (see Appendix C). In his presentation, Dr. Murray discussed the gap in life expectancies found in different parts of the country, global comparisons in life expectancy rates between the United States and other countries, and behavioral risk factors—tobacco, alcohol, obesity, high blood pressure, and blood sugar—that can have a direct impact on life expectancy. Dr. Murray also offered several strategies for future research endeavors and for increasing life expectancies in the United States. Among his suggestions were increasing the availability of county-level data to improve capabilities for monitoring and tracking disparities, developing strategies for framing health disparities concerns that include a greater acceptance of international models, and adopting policies that would foster a broader spectrum of innovation toward reducing health disparities.

Dr. Dolores Acevedo-Garcia offered another perspective in her presentation on the impact of an individual's place of residence on health, discussing how living in disadvantaged metropolitan neighborhoods can have profound developmental, emotional, and physical effects on children and how these effects can have long-term implications throughout an individual's life course. Among other suggestions, she proposed that, rather than working to salvage poverty neighborhoods, children would be better off moving to neighborhoods or areas that are rich with opportunity (such as those with access to healthy foods and safe environments) so they would not have to experience the consequences of living with poverty, crime, and other societal influences.

During the discussion period following the presentations, Roundtable members and sponsors, workshop participants, and attendees discussed concerns and offered strategies for addressing several different factors related to health disparities. Among the topics discussed were the current state of the politics in the United States, the language and framing of disparities, institutional racism, data collection problems, collaborations and community innovations, and efforts toward reducing health disparities in St. Louis. The issues of framing and racism were the subjects that sparked the most lively discussion, with several workshop attendees stressing the importance of creating an open dialogue about these issues and the need for developing strategies to bring all relevant stakeholders together to discuss solutions.

During the afternoon session, Drs. Edward F. Lawlor and Carol Horowitz presented their paper, "Community Approaches to Addressing Health Disparities" (see Appendix D). The paper assesses the implications for developing actionable strategies and describes the benefits of—and approaches to—integrating clinical and community-based approaches to affect communities and reduce health disparities. Dr. Horowitz stressed that hybrid models, which blend clinical and community-based approaches, should integrate community participation and involvement and community ownership into disparities initiatives. Dr. Lawlor suggested that, for any community initiative to succeed, power and sophistication must be developed at the community level for communities to have the knowledge and skills necessary to gather their own social and economic data rather than relying on standard epidemiological data or health indicators alone. In this way, the health status of communities can be evaluated, monitored, and tracked over time. Dr. Lawlor also proposed that communities adopt strategies for leveraging existing public and community partnerships, aligning goals with other stakeholders, and enacting policy changes that redirect their efforts to include a health focus. He believes that strategies such as these would have a dramatic impact on health disparities in the United States.

Following the presentation, workshop participants and attendees shared views concerning leadership, funding, and community capacity, among other issues. While there was some disagreement about whether the infrastructure currently exists to cultivate a new generation of leaders, there was consensus about the importance of committing time and resources to identifying, training, and mentoring individuals in communities who could become future leaders. Although strategies and methodologies varied, workshop presenters and attendees fundamentally agreed that additional, consistent funding was a necessity for community initiatives to succeed, and efforts to partner with relevant stakeholders and existing community-development ventures should be encouraged and actively pursued. Several workshop participants stressed that community initiatives should include community members as active participants in the planning and implementation of a program. In addition, initiatives must include plans for ongoing evaluations to measure and track a program's progress and to strive to be sustainable.

Workshop attendees also had the opportunity to hear from several presenters about their efforts to implement and manage local community interventions, as well as from representatives from the business community who discussed their organizations' efforts to reduce health disparities. Representatives from the Centers for Disease Control and Prevention's (CDC's) Racial and Ethnic Approaches to Community Health (REACH) and Steps to a HealthierUS programs gave individual presentations in which they shared how their community programs were initiated and developed, what some of their challenges have been, and why and how they are experiencing positive results in their communities. Business leaders shared organizational strategies for reducing health disparities and discussed existing challenges and ongoing efforts for reaching future disparities goals.

ORGANIZATION OF THE REPORT

This workshop summary was prepared for the Roundtable membership and includes a collection of presentations and commentary. Sections of the workshop summary not specifically attributed to an individual reflect the views of the rapporteur and not those of the Roundtable on Health Disparities, its sponsors, or the IOM. The contents of the unattributed sections are based on the presentations and discussions at the workshop.

The report is organized into chapters as a topic-by-topic description of the presentations and discussions that took place at the workshop. Its purpose is to present lessons from relevant experience, to delineate a range of pivotal issues and their respective problems, and to offer potential responses as described by workshop participants.

Although this workshop summary provides an account of the individual presentations, it also reflects an important aspect of the Roundtable philosophy. The public workshop functions as a dialogue among representatives from different sectors and presents their beliefs about which areas may merit further attention. The reader should be aware, however, that the material presented here expresses the views and opinions of the individuals participating in the workshop and not the deliberations and conclusions of a formally constituted IOM study committee. These proceedings summarize only what participants stated in the workshop and are not intended to be an exhaustive exploration of the subject matter or a representation of consensus evaluation.

Chapter 2 includes Dr. Murray's presentation of his recent paper, "Eight Americas: Investigating Mortality Disparities Across Races, Counties, and Race-Counties in the United States" (see Appendix C), examining the gap in life expectancies found in different parts of the United States, and Dr. Acevedo-Garcia's presentation discussing the connection between a person's place of residence and subsequent health disparities. Further discussion of these and other related topics raised by workshop attendees following these presentations are summarized in the chapter.

Chapter 3 summarizes presentations by Drs. Carol Horowitz and Edward Lawlor, discussing their paper "Community Approaches to Addressing Health Disparities" (see Appendix D), which assesses the implications for developing actionable strategies and describes the benefits of—and approaches to—integrating clinical and community-based approaches to affecting communities and reducing health disparities. Additional discussion pertaining to this presentation and to other related issues that were raised in reaction to their remarks are also included in the chapter.

Chapter 4 summarizes presentations by individuals who implement interventions in their own communities as part of the CDC's REACH 2010 and Steps to a HealthierUS programs. These representatives shared information about how the community programs were initiated, how programs have developed, what some of the challenges have been, and why and how they are experiencing positive results.

Chapter 5 summarizes presentations by representatives from the business community that discuss successful strategies and programs aimed at reducing health disparities.

Chapter 6 summarizes the salient points from the workshop and provides an overview for strategies to consider while moving forward. Participants' comments pertaining to issues, such as data concerns, the importance of place, framing, racism, education, policy changes, fostering a broader spectrum of innovation, and funding, are summarized here.

This report provides an account of presentations and discussions that took place during the workshop. It bears emphasizing again that the material presented in this and the following chapters represents the views and opinions of individual workshop participants only and is not to be construed as reflective of the deliberations of a formally constituted study committee. It is not intended to be an exhaustive exploration of the subject matter, but rather a contribution to the larger information-gathering efforts of the Roundtable.

2

The Impact of Geography on Health Disparities in the United States: Different Perspectives

Where an individual chooses to live can have a profound effect on their short- and long-term health. "Eight Americas: Investigating Mortality Disparities Across Races, Counties, and Race-Counties in the United States," a paper by Murray et al. (2006), examines the gap in life expectancies found in different parts of the United States in order to more fully elucidate issues related to health disparities in this country. During the public workshop, Dr. Murray presented this paper, along with additional research investigating mortality and causes of death at the local level in the United States. Dr. Acevedo-Garcia further discussed the connection between a person's place of residence and health disparities, focusing her comments on the impacts of living in specific neighborhood settings or metropolitan areas.

Their presentations are recounted here. Other discussion topics and general comments raised during the session by Roundtable members, sponsors, and audience members are included in the Addressing Health Disparities—Different Perspectives section at the end of the chapter. The Murray et al. paper appears in Appendix C.

EIGHT AMERICAS[1]

The Eight Americas presentation is based on analyses of county-level mortality data from the National Center for Health Statistics (NCHS), collected between 1960 and 2001, explained Dr. Murray. Graphic repre-

[1]This section is an edited transcript of Dr. Christopher Murray's remarks at the workshop.

sentations of county-level mortality data from 1997–2001 show how life expectancy rates for men (ranging from age 62.0 to age 80.2) and women (ranging from age 71.8 to age 84.5) vary depending on an individual's county of birth (Figure 2-1). Like a mosaic, the shades depicting different life expectancy rates appear random and unrelated at first; however, further examination reveals that mortality patterns seem to follow specific geographic patterns.

Data comparing county-level life expectancy rates for men and women over time can be examined in several ways. Figure 2-2 shows the standard deviation of the distribution of life expectancy across counties for men and women between 1960 and 2000. Although the lines depicting the standard deviation of county life expectancies for men and women follow similar trajectories, the differences across counties began to steadily increase after 1980.

Similarly, tracking life expectancies for counties in the top and bottom 2.5 percentiles over time for men and women shows a similar result (Figure 2-3). Although the gap in life expectancies for the counties in the top and bottom 2.5 percent of all U.S. counties remained fairly constant from 1960 until around 1980, it has been growing since that time. Among the bottom 2.5 percent of counties, little or no progress in increasing life expectancies has been seen over the past 20 years. In absolute terms, the differentiation in life expectancies in U.S. counties continues to widen.

According to the U.S. national average, and as seen in data from counties that have historically had the highest life expectancies, male life expectancy has been increasing faster than female life expectancy. The counties with the highest life expectancies in the United States are at levels that surpass those seen in Japan, the country with the highest life expectancies globally.

Defining the Eight Americas

In addition to summarizing county-level analysis, *race-counties*—referring to the county of death and the race of the deceased—were analyzed using 5-year moving averages. Life expectancies were calculated for race groups in every county where mortality among members of a certain race was large enough for the analysis. Data show that the range of life expectancies seen in the United States is even larger when comparing race-counties. Life expectancies as low as 58 years of age were calculated for Native Americans in southwestern South Dakota, and Asian women in Bergen County, New Jersey, have average life expectancies reaching 91 years of age. There is no evidence that the magnitude of the gaps is closing.

Further analysis was conducted using the amassed county and race-county data to identify which diseases accounted for the existing mortality

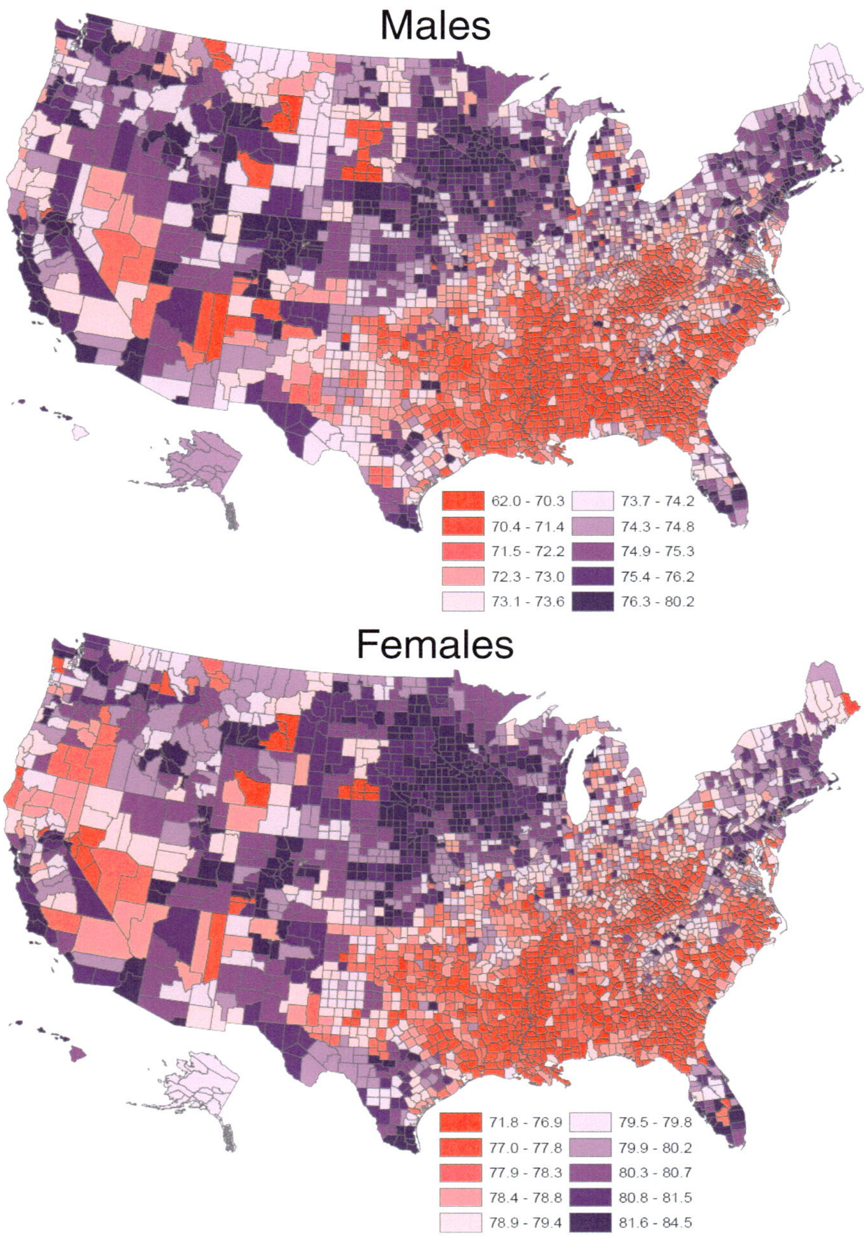

FIGURE 2-1 County life expectancy 1997–2001.

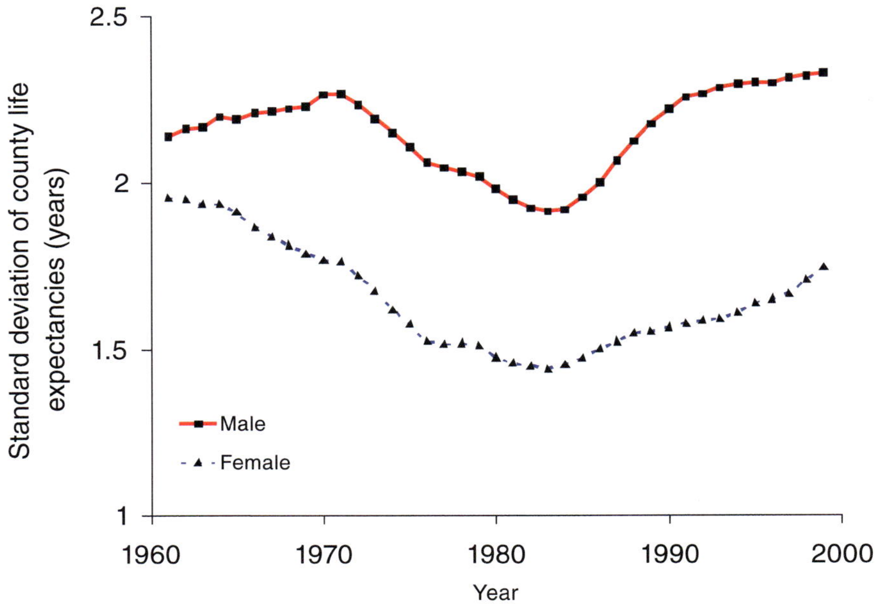

FIGURE 2-2 Width of cross-country distribution of life expectancy.

patterns and the age groups for which the greatest differences in mortality were seen. Using county-level mortality figures proved problematic because they lacked statistical power; too few people were included in the figures from each county to track individual causes of death. The objective in using the new Eight Americas analysis was to identify a discrete number of subgroups, each consisting of a population large enough to statistically analyze mortality by age, sex, and cause. The choice of eight Americas—versus any other number—was to identify a discrete number of subgroups that would have the power to capture most of the broad variation that is seen across counties and race-counties. The Eight Americas are defined in Table 2-1 and represented in Figures 2-4 and 2-5.

Mortality and Cause of Death: Comparisons of the Eight Americas

Using statistical analyses, it is possible to explore life expectancy and causes of death in the Eight Americas. Comparing trends in life expectancy between men and women in the Eight Americas did not show significant changes, indicating on a broad level that disparities are not decreasing and

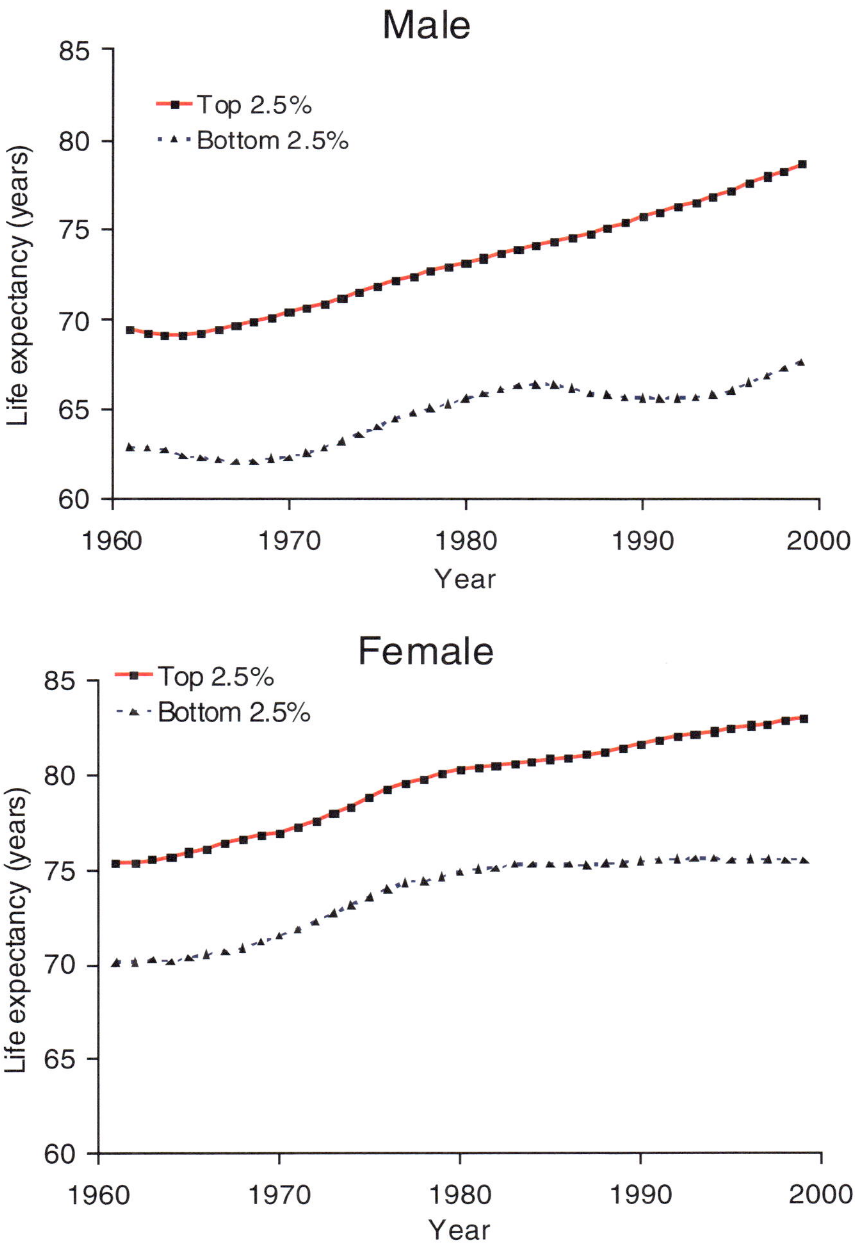

FIGURE 2-3 Life expectancy for top and bottom 2.5 percent of counties.

TABLE 2-1 The Eight Americas

America	General Description	Population (millions)	Average Income Per Capita	Definition
1	Asian	10.4	$21,566	Asians living in counties where Pacific Islanders make up less than 40% of total Asian population
2	Northland low-income rural white	3.6	$17,758	Whites in northern plains and Dakotas with 1990 county-level per capita income below $11,775 and population density less than 100 persons/km^2
3	Middle America	214.0	$24,640	All other whites not included in Americas 2 and 4; Asians not in America 1, and Native Americans not in America 5
4	Low-income whites in Appalachia and the Mississippi Valley	16.6	$16,390	Whites in Appalachia and the Mississippi Valley with 1990 county-level per capita income below $11,775
5	Western Native American	1.0	$10,029	Native American populations in the mountain and plains areas, predominantly on reservations
6	Black Middle America	23.4	$15,412	All other black populations living in counties not included in Americas 7 and 8
7	Southern low-income rural black	5.8	$10,463	Blacks living in counties in Mississippi and the Deep South with population density below 100 persons/km^2; 1990 per capita income below $7,500, and total population size above 1,000 persons (to avoid small numbers)
8	High-risk urban black	7.5	$14,800	Urban populations of more than 150,000 blacks living in counties with cumulative probability of homicide death between 15 and 74 years greater than 1.0%

SOURCE: Adapted from Murray et al. (2006).

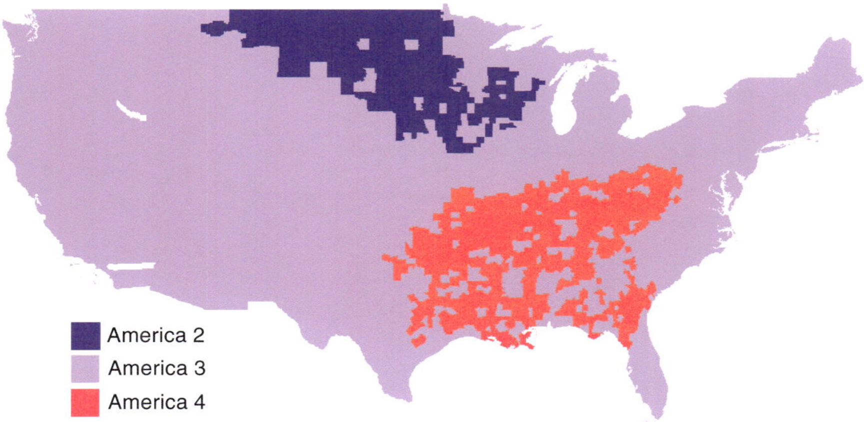

FIGURE 2-4 Americas 2, 3, and 4.

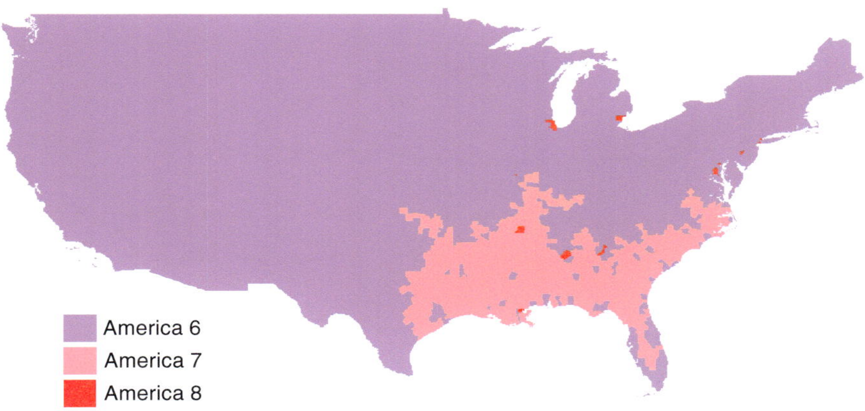

FIGURE 2-5 Americas 6, 7, and 8.

in some cases they are on the rise (see Figure 2-6). However the subtleties found in the graphs do show some interesting patterns in the data.

America One, comprised of Asian Americans living in communities in which Pacific Islanders make up fewer than 40 percent of the total Asian population, has a high life expectancy that continues to increase. America Two shows a dwindling advantage over America Three (Middle America) among men and is showing marked improvement among women. America Four has had a very slow but steady rate of increase. The Appalachian,

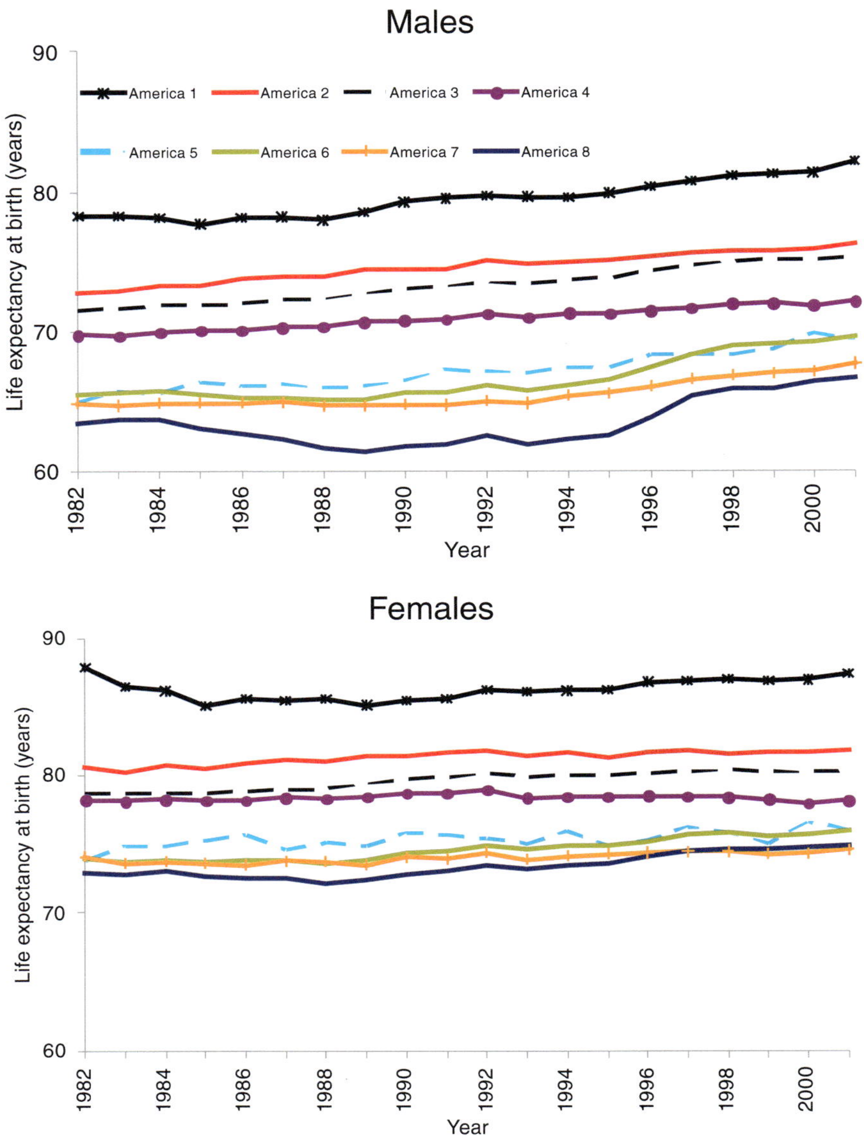

FIGURE 2-6 Life expectancy at birth in the Eight Americas.

Mississippi Valley white populations are increasingly falling behind the rest of white America. Among Native American populations there has been little or no increase in life expectancy for women and moderate increases for men. A similar story holds true for Americas Six and Seven, the African American populations. The large dip in the line depicting life expectancies for men living in America Eight reflects, for the most part, the increase in HIV-related mortality and its subsequent decline. Overall, comparing the graphs for men and women in Americas One through Eight shows that there is very little change in the net effect between the early 1980s and 2000.

County Trends in Life Expectancy

The Eight Americas mortality database contains county-level data dating back to 1960, and an analysis of those data shows a pattern of growing inequalities since 1983. To examine this phenomenon, county-level life expectancy data from 1961 to 1983 were compared with analogous data from 1983 to 1999. Male life expectancy data from 1961 to 1983 (Figure 2-7a) show several areas that have a statistically significant increase in life expectancy greater than the national average; several areas that are equal to or indistinguishable from the national average; and several counties that have life expectancies that are statistically significant below the national average. Counties in red show areas in which there has been no statistically significant decline in life expectancy at the county level for the 22-year time period. Analysis showing life expectancy for men from 1983 to 1999 (Figure 2-7b) shows less progress; there are many more counties with a rate of change that is indistinguishable from zero, and some counties near the Mississippi Valley have life expectancies that dropped. Among women, similar findings are seen when comparisons are made between life expectancy data from 1961 and 1983 (Figure 2-8a); however, data from 1983–1999 show that life expectancy among women in several counties is dropping (Figure 2-8b).

With the exception of the Spanish flu pandemic of 1918 and 1920, there have been constant increases in life expectancy in the United States for more than 100 years, a finding consistent with life expectancy rates seen in other high-income countries. Yet there is a subset of the United States for which life expectancy at the county level for women, in particular, is dropping. This finding is quite unusual in recent mortality history among high-income countries.

To help explain why life expectancy has been decreasing in certain segments of the United States, the cause of death for men and woman, compared by age group, was analyzed using county-level data. Analyses show that, among both men and women, mortality attributable to cardio-

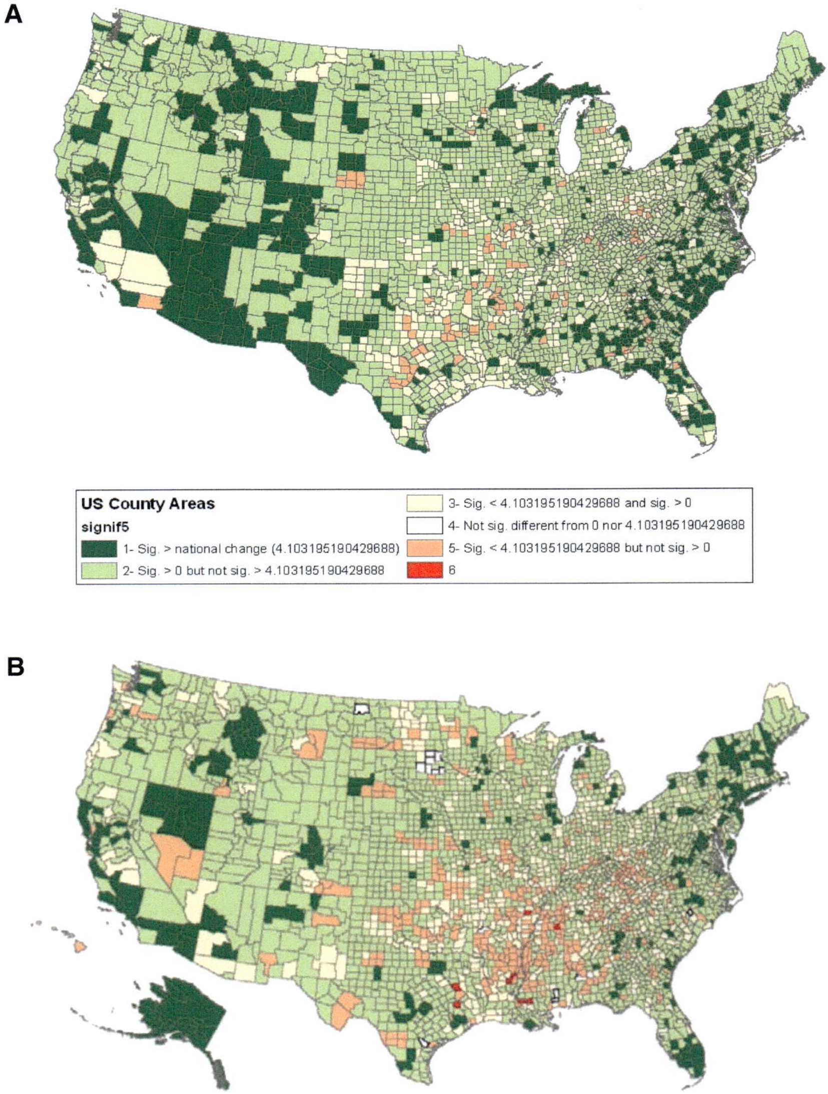

FIGURE 2-7 Change in male life expectancy: (a) 1961–1983, (b) 1983–1999.

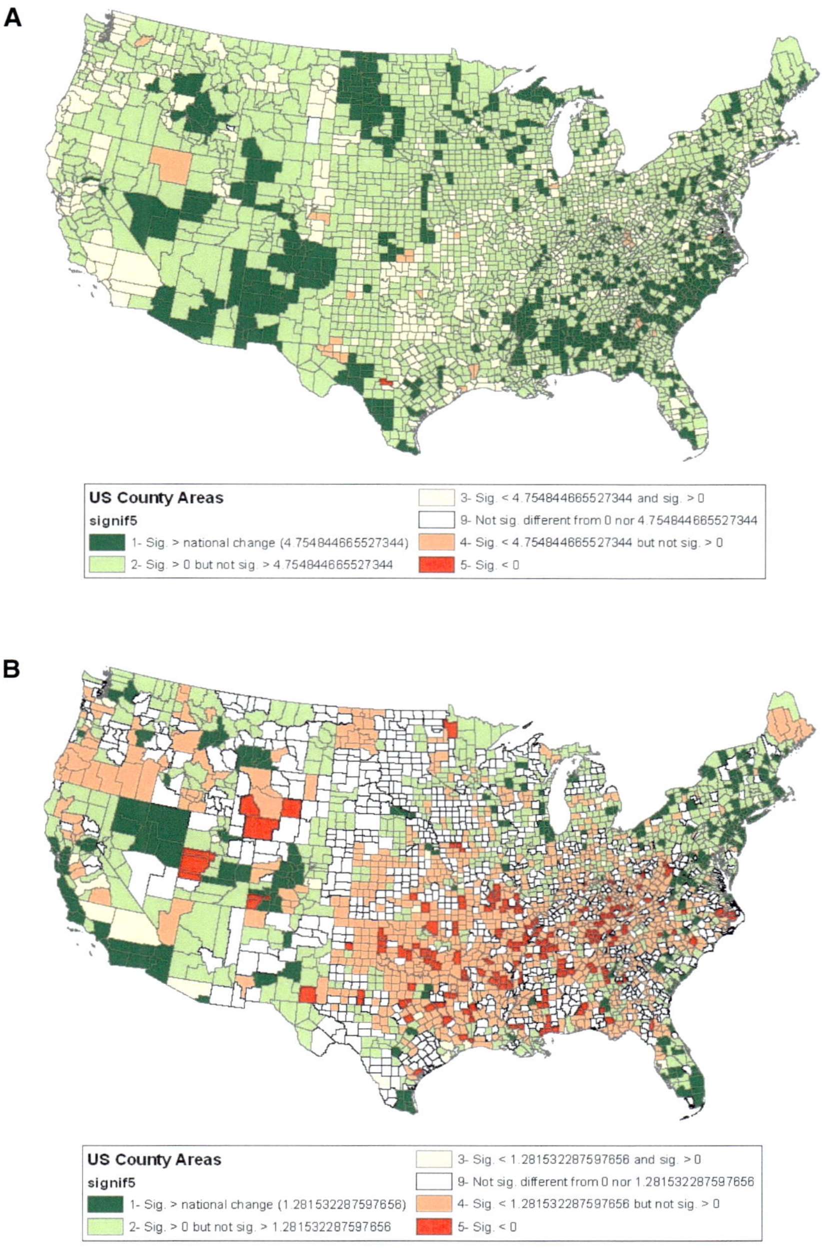

FIGURE 2-8 Change in female life expectancy: (a) 1961–1983, (b) 1983–1999.

vascular disease has been declining steadily at rates that surpass increases in mortality for other noncommunicable diseases. In younger age groups, mortality from HIV, homicide (in men), and lung cancer are evident. However, in the counties in which life expectancy is dropping, cardiovascular disease is actually increasing, unmasking the rise in other causes. It remains to be seen whether the general decline in cardiovascular disease in the United States will result in more counties experiencing a background rise in these other causes of death.

County-level data were also used to examine the relationship between health disparity and wealth to determine whether the gap in poverty levels between counties would match the gap seen in overall health. Income information gleaned from the 2000 census, together with county-level data from the tax return database of the Internal Revenue Service, revealed that while life expectancy in several counties is dropping, the counties with decreasing life expectancies are not getting markedly poorer.

Global Perspective of the Eight Americas

An alternate way to examine the U.S. data is to compare the findings from the Eight Americas with similar data collected from other countries around the globe. Examining the relationship between health disparities and wealth, it becomes evident that other high-income countries are experiencing analogous increases in income levels, yet they are experiencing these changes without health disparities increasing as they are in the United States. Further research must be conducted to investigate why.

The only other countries in which life expectancy has fallen in the past 50 years have been in the former Soviet Union and countries in Eastern and Southern Africa with high HIV prevalence. In the 1930s, some low-income countries experienced a rise in life expectancy, but in the past 50 years this occurrence has been limited to high-income countries. The combination of the Eight Americas' patterns and trends, along with the recent discovery of the subset in the United States in which life expectancy is decreasing, shows that disparities are not getting smaller in the nation and, in fact, there is every expectation that they will continue to grow.

To gain this global perspective, biomedical data representing the cause of death among men from two groups, America One and America Eight, were graphed along with comparable data from Japan, the United Kingdom, Russia, and West Africa (Figure 2-9). Comparisons were made looking at mortality figures for HIV/AIDS, intentional injuries, unintentional injuries, other noncommunicable diseases, other communicable diseases, cardiovascular diseases, and cancers.

Among children ages 0–4 years, mortality in America Eight is much higher than America One and is about equivalent to the Russian Federa-

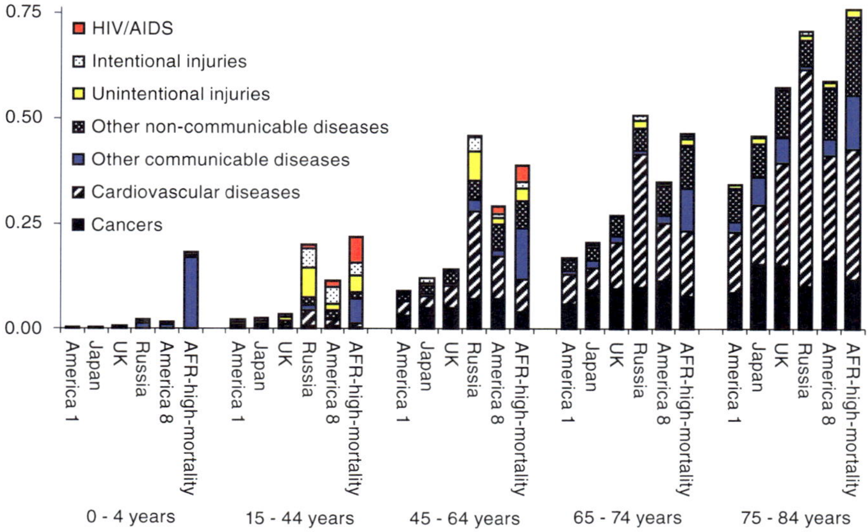

FIGURE 2-9 Male causes of death in the Eight Americas compared to Japan, the United Kingdom, Russia, and West Africa. NOTE: AFR-high-mortality, made up largely of countries in West Africa and excluding countries with very high mortality due to HIV/AIDS.
SOURCE: Murray et al. (2006).

tion. Child mortality in America Eight is almost 10 times lower than in West Africa, meaning that a child living under the harshest conditions in America will still fare considerably better than a child living in West Africa. These findings change dramatically when comparing young high-risk urban black American men to West African men ages 15 to 44, and middle-aged adults ages 45 to 64. In these instances the gap among America Eight, West Africa, and the Russian Federation is not large. In fact, rather than mortality being 10 times lower for individuals in the United States as seen among children 0–4 years of age, mortality among the higher age groups is nearly equivalent. The difference in mortality seen among men cannot be attributed solely to increases in HIV rates. If HIV is not factored in for any of the countries, mortality patterns found in America Eight are still comparable to those found in West Africa. The excess mortality among men is related to communicable and noncommunicable diseases, cardiovascular disease, and to some extent cancers, rather than to homicide and HIV, as might be expected. The mortality pattern for women is very similar.

Another way to examine these data is to compare mortality rates across the Eight Americas with the range found in high-income countries

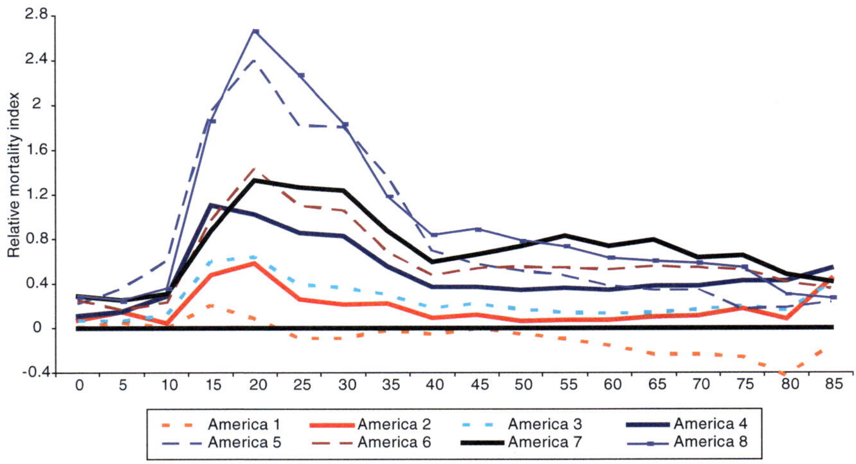

FIGURE 2-10 Mortality in the Eight Americas by age compared to other high-income countries.

(Figure 2-10). The relative mortality index measured on the Y axis ranges from –0.4 to 2.8, meaning that any mortality rate in America for a specific age group is 2.6 times higher (or lower) than the worst of the high-income countries. Therefore, any relative mortality index greater than 1.0 denotes a subgroup in the United States (Americas One to Eight) that fares worse than any other high-income country at the national level. While child mortality rates in the United States compare favorably to those found in other high-income countries, mortality for young and middle-aged adults in Americas Five to Eight fall dramatically behind other high-income countries.

Risk Factors

To investigate what risk factors contribute to biomedical and non-communicable diseases, large databases were sought to provide the necessary input. The National Health and Nutrition Examination Survey (NHANES),[2] typically the best source for biomedical measurements and biomarkers, did not yield sample sizes large enough for the data to be analyzed at the level of the Eight Americas. The Behavioral Risk Factor

[2]In-depth survey compiled by the Centers for Disease Control and Prevention's NCHS that combines in-person interviews with standardized physical examinations, diagnostic procedures, and lab tests with national rather than state representation (NCHS, 2008).

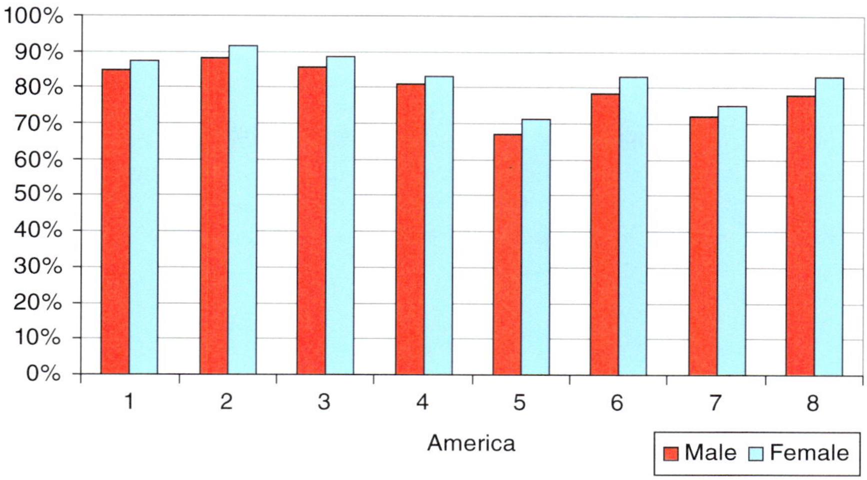

FIGURE 2-11 Difficult-to-explain disparities between Eight Americas on the basis of reported health care access.

Surveillance System (BRFSS)[3] is a rich data source, but it does not provide biomarker information. In order to use the data from the two sources, a method was devised to combine BRFSS and NHANES data to determine how self-reported measures from both data sets were related, and then estimates were calculated for some of the risk factors that require biomarkers. Several interesting observations were made using this method.

BRFSS data were used to examine health plan coverage across the Eight Americas (Figure 2-11). The lowest self-reported health plan coverage was seen in America Five (Western Native Americans); however, this may be an anomaly since health care is provided on reservations in addition to health plan coverage. Slightly lower health plan coverage is also seen in America Seven compared with the other subgroups. Further analyses looking at utilization measured by self-reported data in response to the question "Did you see a doctor or have a check-up in the last twelve months?" failed to show a dramatic gradient in financial access that is strongly related to the disparities seen in the outcomes.

What about behavioral risk factors such as tobacco, diet, or physical activity? The recent World Health Organization's Comparative Risk Assessment (WHO, 2002) work highlighted that the likely candidates for explain-

[3]State-based system of telephone-administered health surveys that collects information on health risk behaviors, preventive health practices, and health care access (BRFSS, 2008).

ing behavioral risk factors in the United States are tobacco, alcohol, obesity, high blood pressure, and blood sugar. Therefore, an attempt was made to quantify these risks across the Eight Americas (Figure 2-12a–e).

Of the major noncommunicable risk factors that are important determinants of health in the United States, obesity, blood sugar, and hypertension appear to be strongly related to the gradients across the Eight Americas. Considerably more work must be done to determine what the net effect of addressing each of those risk factors would have on the differences that are seen across the Eight Americas.

Policy Focus

When considering potential policy implications related to reducing health disparities, it is important to speculate beyond the health insurance debate. In the policy arena there is an assumption that improving financial access would address many of the disparities seen in the United States. However, this is unlikely to be the case although providing financial access would undoubtedly reduce catastrophic spending and result in some improvements in health. A recent Institute of Medicine report (IOM, 2002) enumerated the number of deaths attributable to the lack of health insurance; however, while not inconsequential, the number of deaths attributable to the lack of health insurance would not be comparable to the increase in mortality attributable to health disparities seen across the Eight Americas.

The analysis around the Eight Americas focuses on noncommunicable diseases particularly in young and middle-aged adults. Yet adults in these age groups do not benefit from Medicare and therefore their medical interests are rarely considered in matters relating to public finance or national medical policy. To decrease mortality from noncommunicable diseases, fundamental public health principles would advocate for changes in diet, physical activity, tobacco and alcohol use, and biological risk factors that can be managed through primary care, such as blood pressure, blood sugar, and cholesterol. Can noncommunicable diseases be addressed even more effectively? It seems unlikely, given the experiences of other countries, that one solution will work for the entire U.S. population given the differences across the Eight Americas; both substantively in terms of health patterns and because of cultural variations among different groups. Although there has been considerable attention on reducing health disparities and innumerable public and philanthropic programs have focused on reaching this goal, little success has been made toward decreasing health disparities at the national level.

Dr. Murray believes the appropriate policy response would be to foster a broader spectrum of innovation in addressing both the behavioral risks and the pharmacologically manageable biological risks for noncommunicable disease. It is also essential to have rigorous monitoring and ongoing evaluation when fostering innovation. With these measures in place, successful programs can be recognized, their results can be documented, and the methods can be shared and replicated nationally. This is an appropriate model to follow given how little is known about changing risks—pharmacologically manageable risks and others—at the local level.

By looking at health care from different perspectives, the management of risk factors—blood pressure, cholesterol, and blood sugar—can be evaluated in relation to other existing data sources. NHANES data, for example, show that only 50 percent of hypertensives are being managed, and about 25 percent of people with high cholesterol and about 45 percent of diabetics are being treated. Examining these data in terms of who is receiving appropriate treatment reveals that the number of patients receiving appropriate care dropped to dramatically low levels in terms of outcomes. In a country that spends the most per capita on health care by a large margin, the enormously important risk factors for which there are effective therapies are being managed by only 50 percent of hypertensives. The only way to broaden the reach of effective interventions is through innovations at the local level.

There are many models to investigate for reducing health disparities in the United States. Pay-for-performance models have been proposed, as well as the idea of creating incentives for individuals who receive treatment to reduce their health risk. Conditional cash transfers or financial incentives, for example, could be given for getting blood pressure checked or for managing cholesterol appropriately. A paradigm for this progressive model can be seen in Mexico, where randomized trials looking at conditional cash transfers have shown promise for getting people to use preventive services. While there are no obvious answers for addressing these issues, there are several local innovations that should be tested.

Murray noted that while disparities are increasing in the United States, infant, child, and adult mortality and life expectancy are consistently dropping the ranking of the United States among other countries when health outcomes are compared. Over the last 30 years, the U.S. position in a table of comparable health outcomes has steadily fallen. Alternately, other countries have a rate of improvement that is higher than that of the United States. In conclusion, he observed, it is imperative that the United States adopt an agenda for improving health for Americas Four, Five, Six, Seven, and Eight, as well as the majority of Middle America who are falling behind the rest of the high-income world. Perhaps the answers to addressing health disparities will also have direct relevance for understanding why the United States is falling behind other high-income countries around the world.

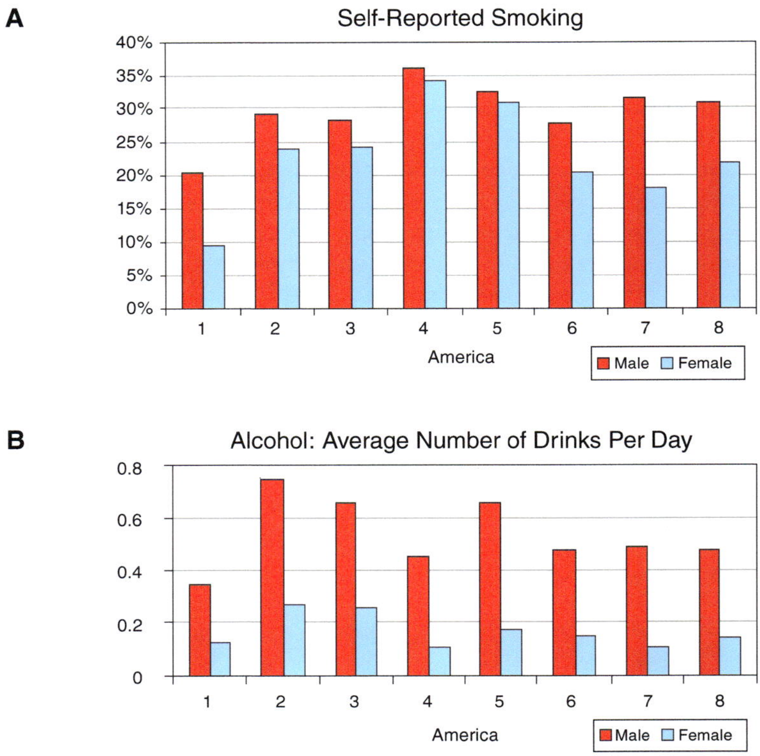

FIGURE 2-12 Quantifying risks across the Eight Americas: (a) Smoking: Tobacco is one of the most important risk factors for health and reducing smoking would markedly improve everybody's health. However, since no clear gradient is seen in the data, decreasing smoking rates may reduce some of the disparities, but ultimately would not have a large affect. (b) Drinks of alcohol per day: America Two, which has the best mortality for white Americans, has the highest average number of drinks per day. Drinks of alcohol per day is an important public health risk factors, but it may not hold the key to understanding the huge gradients across the Americas. (c) Obesity: Obesity data were calculated from BRFSS data corrected for self-report files. For women there is a marked gradient across the Eight Americas in obesity, going up such that Americas 5–8 are greater than 45 percent obese for women and over 30 percent obese for men. Future work will use attributable mortality calculations to examine what the reduction in disparities and life expectancy would be if obesity could be reduced. (d) Uncontrolled hypertension: Substantial gradients exist across the Eight Americas where there are levels of hypertension for women, reaching nearly 30 percent in the bottom Americas 6–8, and a gradient that is smaller, but nevertheless still very substantial for men. (e) Blood sugar: A steady gradient exists, perhaps correlated to the obesity pattern. Blood sugar levels

C

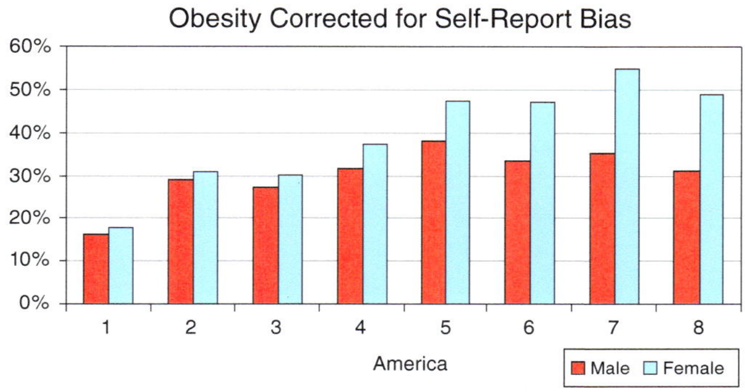

D

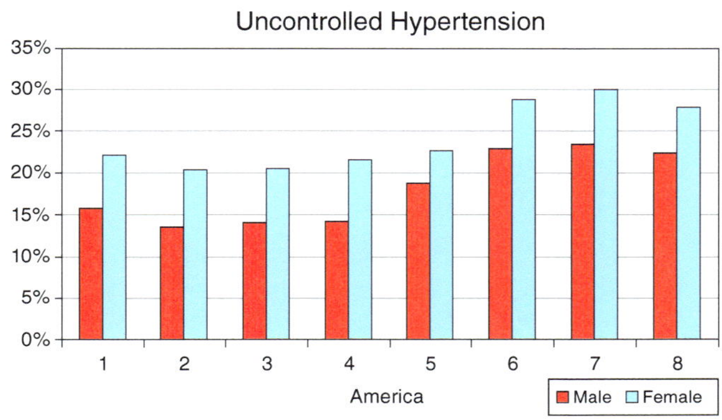

E

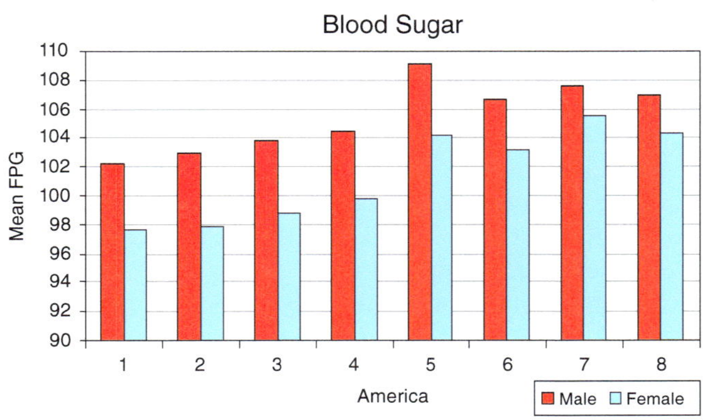

are markedly higher in Native Americans which may be caused in part by a genetic component. Again, the pattern resembles the gradient seen in outcomes across the Eight Americas.

Additional Clarification

Dr. Murray was asked why Hispanics were not included in the Eight Americas, since they represent the largest growing minority group in the United States. He explained that Hispanic Americans were not represented because county-level life expectancy data comparing death certificates and census reports for Hispanic are unreliable; recorded life expectancies in some counties were found to be as high as 190 to 250 years of age. Fundamental differences exist between how Hispanic status gets reported by physicians or relatives on death certificates and self-reported data on the census, and there has been little success in finding a way to reconcile these data sources. Compared with other groups in a similar place or with a similar socioeconomic status, Hispanics seem to have higher life expectancies. This would mean that the white Hispanic population would be comparable to that of America Two. The data for black Hispanic populations are undetermined.

OTHER PERSPECTIVES: THE INFLUENCE OF GEOGRAPHY ON HEALTH DISPARITIES[4]

Where a person resides, or features of a particular area, can have a direct impact on his or her health outcomes and mortality, explained Dr. Acevedo-Garcia in her presentation to the Roundtable. When examining geographic disparities, whether using the geographic boundaries defined in the Eight Americas or using other geographic boundaries, it is important to make connections between those geographies and the social determinants of a health framework. Specific areas should map onto socioeconomic factors driving racial inequality, such as state income inequality or disparities in neighborhood environments in metropolitan areas. The distribution of opportunity across neighborhoods in metropolitan areas can have a profound effect on socioeconomic advancement and health outcomes.

Metropolitan areas are defined as core urban areas—the central city—and the surrounding suburbs. These distinctions are important because housing and labor markets, as well as other factors that shape opportunity in America, operate differently between and across metropolitan areas. The majority of the people in the United States live in metropolitan areas. Two-thirds of all of the children in the United States live in the 100 largest metropolitan areas, and 40 percent (18 of 45 million) of those children live in what are called majority/minority metropolitan areas in which minority children are actually the majority (Acevedo-Garcia et al., 2007). Examples from the 2000 census (Acevedo-Garcia et al., 2007) include the following:

[4]This section is an edited transcript of Dr. Acevedo-Garcia's remarks at the workshop.

- Chicago (2.2 million children; 51% minority [nonwhite])
- Dallas (1 million children; 53% minority [nonwhite])
- Los Angeles (2.7 million children; 80% minority [nonwhite])
- Washington, DC (1.3 million children; 50% minority [nonwhite])

Metropolitan areas have been examined very extensively from an ecological, demographic, and urban planning perspective, because they shape equality in the United States.

Although large disparities are not reflected in U.S. child mortality rates, it is important to focus on children and adolescents because, from a developmental life-course perspective, what happens in childhood is going to impact disease outcomes in adulthood. How opportunity is experienced in metropolitan areas will directly impact the environment in which children live. In turn, this will affect their life course and, subsequently, the long-term economic disparities extant in those metropolitan regions.

Neighborhoods as the Focus of Health Disparities

While to a large extent the nation's health care policy is determined by policies instituted by individual states, research from such disciplines as social epidemiology and human development shows that neighborhoods have an impact on children's health and their developmental outcomes, above and beyond individual- and family-level factors. Poor neighborhood conditions may put children at risk for developmental delays, teen parenthood, and academic failure, resulting in long-term implications throughout the life course. Factors such as access to healthy foods and the safety of the environment will determine a neighborhood's influence on the residents' health. Disadvantaged neighborhood environments are associated with hazardous physical environments, poor-performing schools, and a lack of public safety (Brooks-Gunn et al., 1997). Consistent with the findings of the Eight Americas, research suggests that health and social determinants show large geographic variations in absolute terms and in the level of disparities.

Opportunity-rich neighborhoods do exist in metropolitan areas, but not all children have access to them. Therefore, the neighborhoods to which everyone should aspire already exist in each metropolitan area. The challenge is making those neighborhoods accessible to everyone. Housing markets in metropolitan areas are structured so that there are vast disparities in access to neighborhoods with opportunity. Large disparities in opportunity in metropolitan areas have a substantial impact on the well-being of America's children and, in turn, on economic and social prospects of entire metropolitan regions. Metropolitan areas with better health outcomes and smaller disparities should ideally serve as examples for other communities, and their policies and procedures should be evaluated and replicated in other areas across the nation.

To gain perspective on the variation that exists across metropolitan areas, comparisons were made between rates of low birth weight by ethnicity (Asian, black, Hispanic, and white) for the 100 largest metropolitan areas in the United States for the years 2001–2002 (Figure 2-13) using data from the National Center for Health Statistics Vital Statistics. Low-birth-weight babies, weighing less than 2.5 kilograms at birth, are considered at increased risk for negative health outcomes, including higher rates of infant mortality. The analysis compared low-birth-weight rates ranked from 3 to 6 percent of all births, up to 9 to 12 percent of births in each metropolitan area. According to Healthy People 2010 objectives, the nation should strive for a low-birth-weight rate of 5 percent.

In over 90 percent of metropolitan areas, white children have low-birth-weight rates between 3 and 6 percent, a rate very similar to the distribution of low-birth-weight children among Hispanics. This means that there is not a large disparity when comparing low birth weights between whites and Hispanics. However, there are large disparities between Hispanics and whites when comparing socioeconomic outcomes. Consequently, although significant problems in terms of some health outcomes do not currently exist, the conditions under which Hispanic children are living are deteriorating due to their declining socioeconomic status, and this will predictably and negatively affect outcomes early in their lives. In nearly 70 percent of

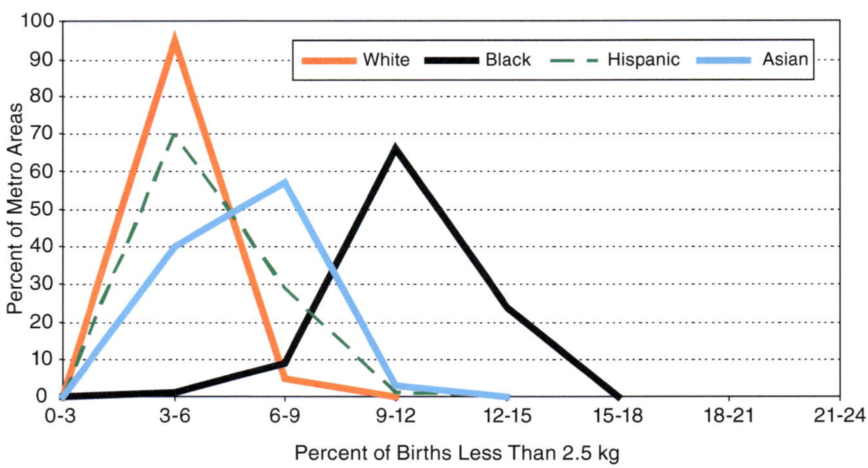

FIGURE 2-13 Low-birth-weight rates: distribution by race/ethnicity.
SOURCE: Dr. Acevedo-Garcia slide presentation.

metropolitan areas, black children have low-birth-weight rates between 9 and 12 percent. Efforts are under way to quantify the differences seen among different racial and ethnic groups, but it should be noted that variations result in entirely different worlds of opportunity and ranges of access to different positive influences and experiences in metropolitan areas. Asian children generally cluster closely to the white children in the best possible part of the distribution. This finding mirrors the findings of Dr. Murray's research.

If one were to graph a theoretical equal representation of poverty rates for neighborhoods in a metropolitan area, the distribution would be similar to that seen in Figure 2-14a. Research has shown that residing in neighborhoods with 20–40 percent poverty rates can impact child development (Brooks-Gunn et al., 1997). If this hypothetical distribution existed, less than 10 percent of all children would live in neighborhoods in which poverty rates exceed 40 percent. There would also be a comparable distribution of black and white children. This is a theoretical metropolitan area that is not found anywhere.

In the Chicago metropolitan area, fewer than 25 percent of all black children live in neighborhoods with low poverty rates between 0–10 percent; the remainder lives in neighborhoods with poverty rates between 10.1 and 40 percent (Figure 2-14b). In contrast, over 85 percent of white children living in the Chicago metropolitan area live in neighborhoods with poverty rates below 10.1 percent, and the majority of the remaining children live in areas with poverty rates ≤20 percent. There is very little overlap between the distributions of neighborhood quality for white children and black children. Opportunity neighborhoods exist for white children, but, on the whole, black children live in totally different neighborhoods.

The distribution of neighborhood quality is not solely dictated by a family's socioeconomic status. Comparing the distribution of poor black children with poor white children in Chicago (Figure 2-14c) shows that less than 5 percent of poor black children live in low-poverty neighborhoods, and more than 95 percent live in high-poverty neighborhoods (Acevedo-Garcia et al., 2007). Black families, even those with a higher income, tend to live in high-poverty neighborhoods, while white families with lower incomes are more likely to live in higher income neighborhoods. Nearly 75 percent of poor white children live in neighborhoods in which the poverty level is ≤10 percent. This means that white children do not live in areas in which they have to contend with familial and environmental pressures associated with living in high-poverty neighborhoods.

When the poverty composition of neighborhoods is analyzed by comparing nonpoor black children to poor white children, the distribution of poor white children remains more favorable than the distribution for nonpoor black children (Figure 2-14d). This finding is consistent with

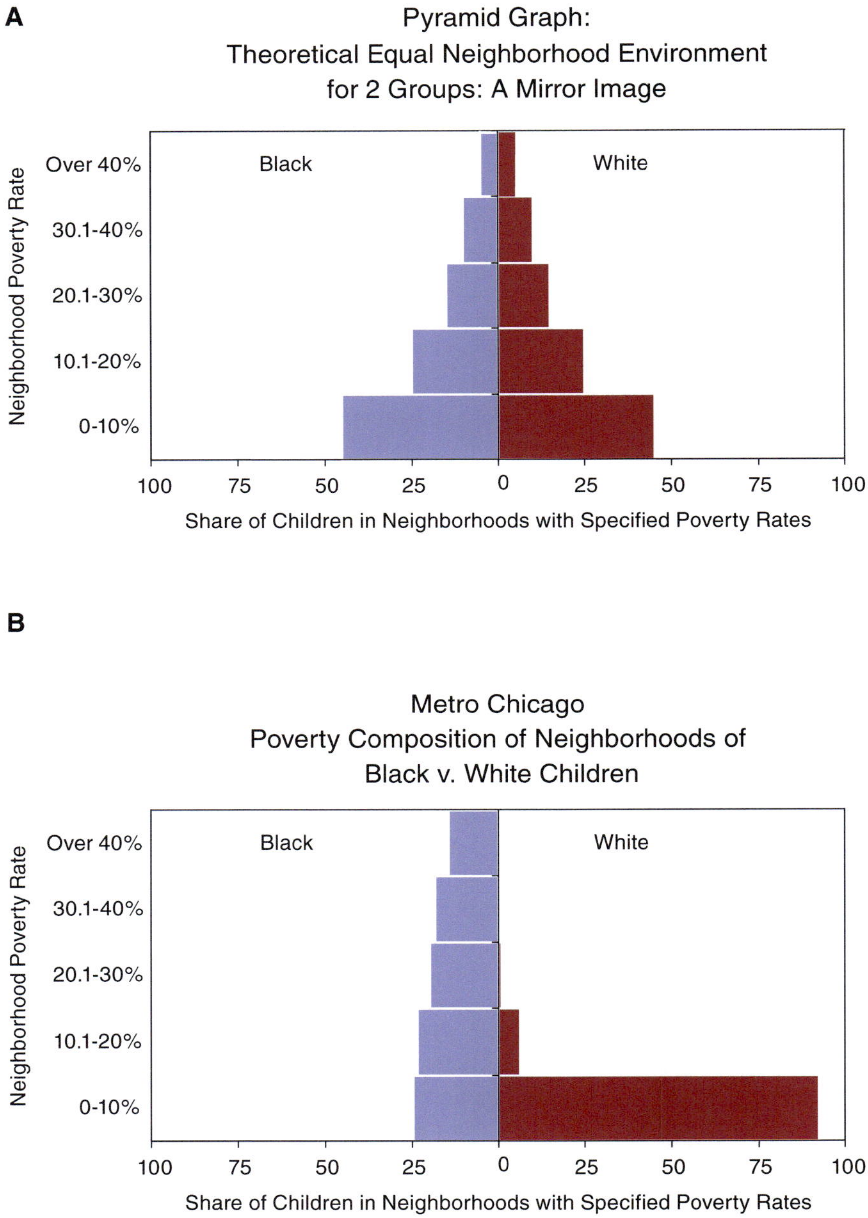

FIGURE 2-14a–d Distribution of poverty rates for neighborhoods in a metropolitan area.

C

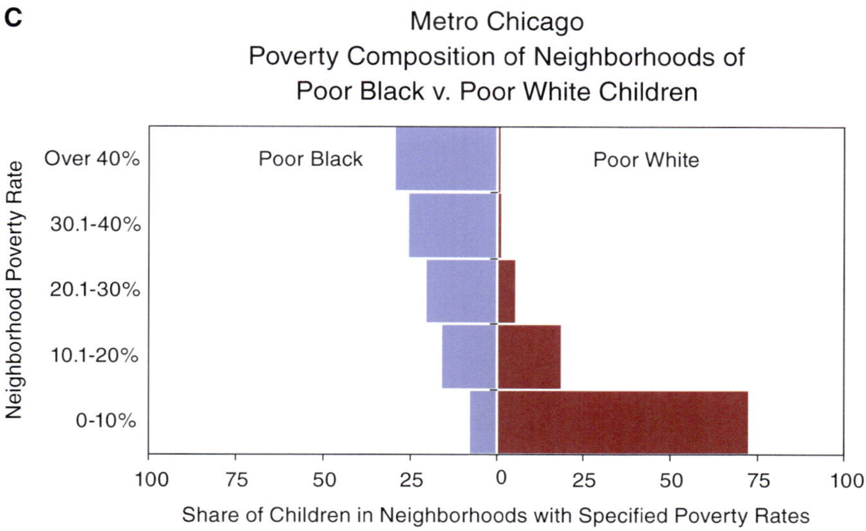
Metro Chicago
Poverty Composition of Neighborhoods of
Poor Black v. Poor White Children
Neighborhood Poverty Rate
Over 40%
30.1-40%
20.1-30%
10.1-20%
0-10%
Poor Black
Poor White
100
75
50
25
0
25
50
75
100
Share of Children in Neighborhoods with Specified Poverty Rates

D

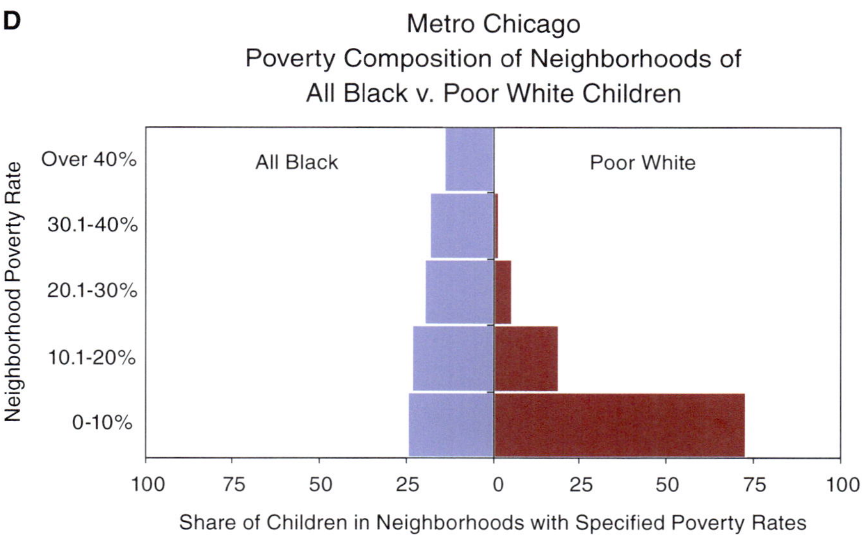
Metro Chicago
Poverty Composition of Neighborhoods of
All Black v. Poor White Children
Neighborhood Poverty Rate
Over 40%
30.1-40%
20.1-30%
10.1-20%
0-10%
All Black
Poor White
100
75
50
25
0
25
50
75
100
Share of Children in Neighborhoods with Specified Poverty Rates

distributions from other metropolitan cities that were analyzed. When analyses were done comparing neighborhood poverty rates for black, white, and Hispanic children living in the 100 largest U.S. metropolitan areas in 2000, it was evident that black and Hispanic children consistently live in neighborhoods with much higher poverty rates than white children. In fact, the socioeconomic profile for Hispanic children at the family, neighborhood, and school levels is similar to the profile of black children. If Hispanic children continue to live in these high-poverty environments, outcomes for Hispanic children will eventually resemble the outcomes seen for black children in similar neighborhoods. The long-term implications of this should be considered, stressed Dr. Acevedo-Garcia, especially in light of the fact that Hispanics are the largest minority group.

Using economic indicators compiled from the 100 largest metropolitan areas, the best and worst neighborhood environments for black, white, Hispanic, and Asian children were identified. Additional analyses were done to determine the worst neighborhoods as far as disparities for Asian, black, and Hispanic children compared with white children (see Table 2-2). In the areas designated as having the worst disparities for black children, the share of black children living in low-income neighborhoods was more than 10 times larger than the share of white children living in low-income neighborhoods.

TABLE 2-2 Best and Worst Neighborhoods from the 100 Largest Metropolitan Areas

Race/Ethnicity	Best Neighborhood Environments	Worst Neighborhood Environments	**Neighborhoods with the Worst Disparities Compared to Whites**
Asian	Austin, TX Baltimore, MD Washington, DC	Bakersfield, CA Fresno, CA New York, NY	Milwaukee-Wausheka, WI Minneapolis-St. Paul, MN
Black	Denver, CO Colorado Springs, CO Raleigh-Durham-Chapel Hill, NC	Buffalo, NY Chicago, IL New York, NY	Mobile, AL Detroit, MI Chicago, IL
Hispanic	Ann Arbor, MI Cincinnati, OH Washington, DC	Bakersfield, CA Providence, RI Springfield, MA	Chicago, IL Hartford, CT Milwaukee-Wausheka, WI
White	Ann Arbor, MI Boston, MA San Francisco, CA	Bakersfield, CA El Paso, TX New York, NY	

Availability and access to health insurance can have a dramatic impact on people in different minority groups, especially for Hispanics. Hispanics are uninsured at rates that surpass other ethnic groups, and there are national and state policies currently in place that limit the access of Hispanics to some services. One example of this was recently seen during discussions of the State Children's Health Insurance Program reauthorization, when coverage for illegal immigrant children was highly debated and eventually defeated. Policies such as these restrict access to health care for immigrant children, a group among which Hispanic children are the majority. The impact of health insurance can also be seen when this issue is analyzed with a regional or local focus.

The Relationship Between Geography and Policy

It is important consider whether health inequities identified between geographic areas can be rectified through policy change. When analyzing geographies areas, geographic entities should be identified that are actionable from a political and policy standpoint. Since political and policy systems in the United States are structured geographically, finding actionable solutions to health disparities and other disparities can be extremely challenging. Patterns of devolution to the states in significant areas of social policy result in, for example, large variations in state child welfare policies. The variations prevent convergence to uniform policies and impede efforts to reduce disparities. Political fragmentation in metropolitan areas also makes disparities issues very difficult to address.

There is a need for socioeconomic interventions and public health or medical interventions, continued Dr. Acevedo-Garcia. Additional research is needed to determine how disparities can be reduced using both types of interventions. In the current political climate, instituting race-based solutions is going to be increasingly more difficult. The Supreme Court recently ruled against school integration programs, and other race-based initiatives are being challenged. For these reasons, it will be necessary to find new frameworks for looking at disparities. If the geography for opportunity framework was to be used and children were redistributed using indicators of opportunity only, the result would be a racially integrated society. Creative strategies such as these must be developed for addressing racially focused issues when efforts to enact policy changes are stymied by political inaction or a lack of political will.

Policies to reduce residential segregation include expanding neighborhood choice in the Department of Housing and Urban Development Section 8 Voucher Program, fair housing enforcement, inclusionary zoning, and increased availability of rental housing. If availability of rental housing is restricted or there are restrictions on density for certain areas, minority households are directly affected because Hispanic and black Americans are disproportionately renters rather than homeowners. Even poor whites have a greater likelihood of being homeowners compared with minorities because of the unequal distribution of wealth and the propensity for white Americans to benefit from intergenerational bequests.

In the housing policy arena, people are very much at ease with discussing place-based approaches versus people-based approaches, intervening in disadvantaged neighborhoods versus moving people from failing neighborhoods into better neighborhoods. Organizations such as the Brookings Institution or the Urban Institute contend that the nation has to do both. The majority of public health professionals have traditionally favored approaches that focus on improving disadvantaged neighborhoods, rather than moving people to new neighborhoods, but it is extremely challenging to try to improve neighborhoods with high poverty rates. Some economic interventions can make a difference, but the problems that exist in these neighborhoods are deeply entrenched and interconnected. Schools, for example, are integral to the neighborhoods, and improving schools can improve neighborhoods to an extent. Yet fixing one facet of a failing neighborhood does not guarantee that success and prosperity will follow.

Baltimore is embarking on a program that has moved about 1,000 families out of the inner city and into the suburbs; 1,000 additional families are waiting to move. The program aims to provide education, employment, and health services to ensure that the move to the suburbs will be successful. Programs such as these show great promise.

To address issues related to health, more researchers have been focusing on disparities among children, and there is now a great deal of evidence showing that brain development has a significant impact later in life, especially involving cognitive development (IOM, 2000). Not addressing disparities may have serious socioeconomic implications. Hispanics play a very significant part in the growth of the workforce, especially among the low-wage workforce. Overall productivity could be affected if these issues are not adequately addressed.

Targeting children is beneficial because they are disproportionately minorities, compared with the U.S. population. The fact that the nation has younger age distributions for minorities than for whites means that going forward there will be greater reliance on minorities to finance the way people live, including who is going to be working and who is going to be paying for Social Security and so on. This needs to be emphasized, because the moral issues are not going to be compelling enough to foster change.

Additional Clarification

Dr. Escarce questioned whether children's access to quality education was more highly correlated with the findings that were shown in Dr. Acevedo-Garcia's presentation rather than issues regarding racial segregation. In response, Dr. Acevedo-Garcia explained that the school data mimicked the patterns seen in the neighborhood data. This would be expected, she believed, since schools are neighborhood-based in the United States. Any kind of segregation and socioeconomic inequalities that exist at the neighborhood level would be translated into the school systems. Hispanic and black children who are disproportionately likely to be poor because their families are poor and live in poor neighborhoods are also going to be disproportionately likely to go to poor schools. Dr. Acevedo-Garcia referred to this as a system of triple jeopardy—poor neighborhoods, poor families, poor schools—and stressed that this composite of problems was one facet of disparities that needs to be addressed.

Dr. Escarce also pointed out that most of Dr. Acevedo-Garcia's solutions, such as rental housing and Section 8, could be construed as trying to improve the way the housing market works. Furthermore, he noted that a great deal of the problem is actually race-based, not socioeconomically based, and that Dr. Acevedo-Garcia's own data would show that the vast majority of white children who are poor do not live in communities in which a lot of people are poor. Even if one could decrease racial segregation and give more minority children better opportunities, the number of children who could be affected would be quite limited. All of the minority kids who are living in very poor neighborhoods could not be moved to other communities.

In response, Dr. Acevedo-Garcia discussed the intervention in Baltimore. To settle a desegregation lawsuit, the courts have proposed that African American residents who choose to participate will be moved from public housing projects in Baltimore City to the suburbs of Baltimore. This is a regional initiative focused on moving people to more affluent suburban areas. Meetings have been held with the program coordinators to determine how to integrate a health component into the program to ensure that people who move to the suburbs do not lose their health care coverage and to make certain that people who move have access to everything they need. However, it has been very difficult to get the sponsoring foundations to focus on adding a health component to their housing initiative. It is important to recognize that funding initiatives that are intersectorial tend to be unpopular, and people lack incentives to work on things that combine more than one sector.

Dr. Acevedo-Garcia also stressed that there is a great deal of evidence showing that early childhood programs, more ambitious than Head Start, are needed to try to eliminate some of the inequalities among children. Another solution would be to move children to better neighborhoods so that, ultimately, fewer expensive public health interventions or early childhood education programs would be required.

In response, Dr. Escarce commented that programs such as these seem unlikely to happen politically, although he agreed that this was probably the only feasible approach for children. New York has a similar program in which small high schools are being created in communities. He also mentioned programs funded by the Bill and Melinda Gates Foundation and their investment in the Global Alliance for Vaccines and Immunization (GAVI). As described by Dr. Murray, GAVI was created as a public–private partnership through a grant from the Bill and Melinda Gates Foundation, to find a way to increase immunization rates using local innovation. The Global Alliance asked countries to apply and propose how they were going to raise childhood immunization; it did not say how they should do it. They simply said that after three years they would pay $20 for every child who is immunized.

In order to develop programs to alleviate health disparities, explained Dr. Escarce, it will be necessary to stop trying to decide whether problems are caused by social determinants or whether or not they are public health problems. There is need to move beyond descriptive academic analyses to testing innovative solutions. There needs to be a national fund for innovative health improvement that has the same attributes that GAVI has shown will work. A public–private partnership, a large pool of resources, local applications, payment for progress, and a strongly embedded monitoring and evaluation program are all necessary in order to learn what is working, continued Dr. Escarce. Further academic debate is also very useful and important to make a shift from describing the inequalities that either stabilize or grow to actually narrowing them. The only way to accomplish this is to take models that foster innovation and subject them to rigorous assessment.

ADDRESSING HEALTH DISPARITIES—DIFFERENT PERSPECTIVES[5]

Reaction to the discussions regarding the relationship between health disparities and geography was thoughtful and, at times, passionate. Several of the issues discussed by the panelists and audience members—the current state of politics in the United States, language and framing, institutional racism, data collection problems, collaborations and community innovations, and health disparities approaches in St. Louis—are detailed here.

---

[5]The following discussions were edited and organized around major themes to provide a more readable summary and to eliminate duplication of topics.

Health Disparities and U.S. Politics

Several audience members shared concerns about the difficulty of addressing health disparities concerns in the current political environment. President Bush plans to veto a bipartisan bill that would enhance coverage for young people and improve access to basic health care, commented Dr. Suggs, because it would be a step toward what President Bush referred to as socialized medicine. However, in Dr. Suggs' opinion, this kind of context to discuss problems inhibits the opportunity to find satisfactory conclusions or remedies. Using a highly charged term like "socialized medicine" polarizes the issue and refocuses the debate to one of ideology rather than finding appropriate solutions to complex issues such as health care reform. Some of the problems that are being dealt with could benefit from a more open, objective, and candid discussion, continued Dr. Suggs. For example, if socialized medicine is untenable, then how can the programs that are in place for elected officials in Congress, for members of the U.S. military through the Department of Veterans Affairs, or, to some extent, for people who benefit from Medicare or Medicaid be rationalized?

Today's burgeoning health care costs have a tremendous effect on society and on general access to quality health care, Dr. Suggs continued. Having power and wealth concentrated among a few industries, such as the pharmaceutical industry and the professional health care industry, can make it difficult to try to enact the reforms necessary to alleviate health disparities in the United States. Medical advancements have increased life expectancies and led to medical interventions that save lives. This also means that individuals who may have died from an illness in years past, can now lead long lives with the aid of hospice or long-term medical care. Yet a disproportionate percentage of people needing these long-term health care options are not protected by the health care policies that are in place today, stated Dr. Suggs. Alternatively, there are people who benefit from the current system without having paid into it. When my mother was growing up as a poor black woman in Mississippi, Dr. Suggs said, the actuary said that she would be dead by the time she was 50 years old. Therefore, when the Social Security system was put into place, it did not include my mother. My mother is now 94 years old and has, in a sense, been a beneficiary of a program that was never intended for black people. This example demonstrates some if the unintended consequences that occur when people who shape public policy ignore the problems related to disparities, concluded Dr. Suggs.

When a pronouncement is made that universal health insurance alone is not enough, it should be expressed with the caveat that people should not step back from advocating for universal coverage, commented another audience member. People need to abandon the notion that health insurance is unnecessary because emergency room care is accessible to everyone. It is important to continue to advocate for insurance, but simultaneously to convince people that an insurance plan or universal coverage alone is not enough, he continued. The health industry in the United States should be based on a foundation of ensuring good health rather than administering sick care as it does now. True health care would take up issues like housing, healthy environments, employment, and income disparities. These are the important things that impact people's lives.

Many health issues are not going to have simple, clinical, insurable interventions, added another member of the audience. Consideration should be given to the environment in which people live and the effects of the choices that people are able to make given the options that they have available. This would ideally lead to a general population approach that, along with changes to insurance policies, could help ensure that people are healthier and, ultimately, that maintaining good health would be less costly.

Framing Health Disparity Issues for a Broader Audience

Several workshop participants were concerned with finding a way to discuss or frame issues related to health disparities in a way that will resonate with policy makers and government workers, and also to capture the public's attention, both locally and nationally.

Fifty years ago the world adopted national income and product accounting, such that the field of macroeconomics was created, explained Dr. Murray. After World War II, people started benchmarking income per capita, and the annual growth rate at income per capita became a central policy target. In the 1970s, when Japan had a higher income growth rate than the United States, it had an incredible affect on the media, the American public, and the U.S. policy debate, continued Dr. Murray. People were very concerned about why the Japanese were pulling ahead of the United States. What is needed now is a situation in which the American public focuses on why the nation is falling behind other high-income countries in terms of health.

Dr. Levi added that an abundance of data suggests that neither politicians nor the American public like hearing or admitting that another country's systems or programs are superior. Americans want an American solution; embracing a French solution or a Canadian solution is not something that resonates. The challenge is to find a way to frame health disparities issues in this country so that people recognize that a problem exists, but to do so without making comparisons that could make people feel that the American way is inferior or that the proposed approach may not be a uniquely American approach. Dr. Lurie added that there is a great deal to learn from less developed countries as well as developed countries.

Framing issues related to health disparities is extremely hard to do in this country, added Dr. Murray, because when you focus on health outcomes, you get one of four apologies. The first apology is that the United States is more diverse than other countries, as if diversity is a sort of scourge that makes it impossible for all residents to be healthy. Even if this argument were taken seriously, it cannot explain why the trends are not very good for the United States. The second and third apologies are that the health problems are caused by HIV or homicide, but it can be easily demonstrated that this is not true. The fourth apology is that it is a lack of insurance. Although that is a component of the problem, the entire issue is much more complex.

The solution to framing issues related to health disparities is to shift from benchmarking health problems to benchmarking the coverage or by tracking care, continued Dr. Murray. This causes the argument to shift from saying that the United States has really bad outcomes and obesity is getting worse, for example, to determining what fraction of Americans or Missourians or people in the Mississippi delta are getting appropriate management of their diabetes. What fractions of those people are receiving appropriate interventions focused on diet or physical activity? If analyses show what is happening and provide comparisons from other settings, either nationally or internationally, it is very difficult to shift the onus of responsibility for those types of performance measures to somebody else.

Ms. Glover Blackwell agreed that it is important to find the appropriate language because the way in which disparities are discussed will determine whether or not there will ever be the political and public will to be able to eliminate disparities. It is also important to try to identify what is making a difference, what is working. At PolicyLink, she explained, we invest in learning how to frame something and how to talk about and understand why it is important to invest in framing. We rarely think that, once we have figured out what needs to happen, there is a need to go out and start a new initiative, because there are so many programs out there already. Yet if we could determine which programs are truly the most successful, we could lift up what works. After lifting up what works, we could determine the elements that make it work. Once the successful elements are identified, those elements could be infused into policy so that the original programs can be expanded and copied. Framing is absolutely important.

She went on: it is also important to join with other people in this country who are committed to trying to transform society so that everybody can participate and everybody can prosper. This is a movement, which is comprised of many people working toward similar goals. Some of these people are in politics or working on housing issues. Some of them are working in environmental health, and some of them are in the workforce. We have to figure out how to join all of these people together.

When legitimate discussions about some of these difficult issues do not take place, the issues sometimes get obscured because ideology keeps people who have vested interests from making necessary changes, commented Dr. Suggs. It makes it impossible to have the kind of honest and open discussions that will be necessary to address issues related to health disparities. It is, after all, a very daunting problem that needs a more aggressive kind of approach.

Ms. Boyce spoke about the power of words. She said: there are concepts I cannot abide and one of them is evidence-based practice. If we knew what evidence was going to work, we would not have health disparities. Evidence-based practice has been used to exclude community-based agencies from funding. Another concept that should be changed is data-driven decision making, when we know that the existing available data are faulty and that individuals are looking at the data disproportionately because of disparities. The words that are being used to describe the system do not match what is really going on in the communities.

In addition, existing policies do not match what needs to happen in communities, continued Ms. Boyce. People are talking about paradigm shifts, and we keep searching for the words to define something different that needs to happen. Dr. Murray said that there needs to be a large pool of money to fund innovation and that only then will the system help us legitimize what works and what will make a difference. But can new words or concepts be coined that will better mirror what needs to happen? Otherwise, we are going to keep using words like "evidence-based practice" and the people who need to be funded will never get the money, because the words that are used for awarding grants and justifying that a program is successful do not fit reality.

Most of us were motivated to come here because we view access to quality health care as a human right, commented Dr. Rhee. The health movement that we are talking about here today mirrors the history of the Civil Rights Movement. As I reflect on my own experience as a physician and medical director and the language that I have been trained to use, I realize that the language I use gives me a lot of power in my community, Dr. Rhee continued. In the world of clinical care, we talk much more about survival, rather than viability. We focus on disease and not wellness. Our emphasis is on immediate gratification or using pills to fix things. We do not necessarily track many of the value kind of outcomes that are really important.

It is important to recognize that language is a major part of the power that we as health care providers wield, continued Dr. Rhee. Nearly 20 percent of gross national product will soon be devoted to health care. Yet the focus of medicine has been on the bench side or bedside, rather than on the curbside (in the community). Ultimately, when you are talking about health disparities improvements, it really is about the curbside interventions and whether or not they work.

Framing Issues About Race and Institutional Racism

The topics of racism and institutional racism spurred a great deal of discussion and debate. It is challenging to find a way to talk about something that causes so many people to recoil, explained Ms. Glover Blackwell. However, race problems will not be solved if we do not talk about them. There must also be recognition that this is a charged discussion that cannot be approached in a way that isolates, accuses, or causes people to want to stay away. The challenge is finding appropriate language to frame the discussion, while also understanding that we have to call it what it is.

Dr. Rhee suggested that the terminology used to discuss these issues must strike a balance. The term "health disparities" might not resonate with the public, but terms such as "racism" or "institutionalized racism" can be very powerful. The language that is used must be forceful and specific, yet it should not cause people to disengage or make them unwilling to join in the discussion to find resolutions.

There is great opposition to changing the status quo, stated Dr. Suggs. Racism is not going to be eliminated using the kind of arguments presented today. Some people are increasingly marginalized on the basis of race or social class and the price that society has to pay for that is enormous. Racial disparities are a disgrace, but they are also enormously expensive for the country. Our discussions should not simply focus on the injustice that health disparities cause, but also consider that it is terribly inefficient and costly if large segments of the population are ignored.

Ms. Wright shared her belief that the message about institutional racism must be targeted to specific audiences, because the variations between audiences can be quite significant. There are multiple approaches to having a constructive dialogue and to bring more people into the conversation in a meaningful way.

Ms. Schwartz noted that all races and ethnicity are going to have to pay attention to this problem because the demographics in this country are changing so rapidly. It used to be that New Jersey was the most diverse state in the country; there was parity in the ratio of African Americans and Hispanics. Today New Jersey is losing citizens, and the only source of new residents is through immigration. These trends are going to drive all of these issues and attention should be paid, because these issues are going to impact everyone.

Dr. Bracho shared her belief that it would be dangerous to talk about geography without highlighting issues regarding poverty and race. Clinical workers and public health professionals must talk about these issues and develop solutions for reducing disparities. The link between poverty and disparities, and racism and disparities has been established. Yet little is being done because health disparities are not on the national political agenda.

Dr. Suggs added that there are some issues that need to be discussed regarding the relationship between blacks and Hispanics. Had blacks and poor whites been able to come together in the 1960s and form an effective political coalition, the course of this nation may have changed. Today there is a similar opportunity. If Hispanics and blacks, the largest growing minority and the established minority in this society, respectively, could join together and form an effective coalition focused on addressing the problems of their collective communities, their political clout would be enormous and effective change might be realized.

A member of the audience responded that there have been times during this country's history when disparate groups have successfully joined forces for the greater good, and these efforts significantly changed the political scene both at the time and into the future. People should look for lessons in the annals of history. It is also very important to begin to tie similar issues together, so that people do not think in terms of one isolated problem. Especially in health care, people should merge issues together and work to see the connections between disparate problems.

Data Concerns

Many of the workshop participants expressed concerns about issues related to data accessibility. According to Dr. Murray, his analysis would have gone beyond 2001; however, NCHS stopped releasing data from subsequent years, citing privacy concerns. Yet, continued Dr. Murray, because the NCHS data originate from death certificates that are in the public domain at the local level, this seems peculiar. Since NCHS collects and tabulates data from documents that are in the public domain, it stands to reason that these data should be available to the public. Despite multiple requests to NCHS, the county-level death files have not been made available, stated Dr. Murray. He surmises that it will require pressure on NCHS from policy makers in Washington in order to make the agency reverse its current policy. In any event, he concluded, it is impossible to continue monitoring disparities at the local level unless this policy is reversed.

Dr. Acevedo-Garcia agreed that the lack of data makes her work more challenging and expressed frustration that county data on mortality were no longer available. The county-level data are essential for tracking disparities in the United States, she explained. Although disparities are apparent in the metropolitan-area data, no health surveys are specifically representative of people living in metropolitan areas. Similarly, surveys done at the county, state, and national level are not structured in a way that adequately captures data on health disparity, opportunity, or inequality by geographic region.

Dr. Acevedo-Garcia believes that her greatest challenge will be to conduct simulation work. Her group is planning to combine empirical estimates of neighborhood effects on health with analyses of census data to try to simulate what the impact of policy changes would be on metropolitan areas. These analyses, based on estimates on neighborhood effects on health, would look at such issues as the availability of rental housing to see how this could impact residential segregation and, in turn, how this change would affect some child health outcomes. This kind of simulation work is very hard to do, she said, because it is based on quite a few assumptions. Yet it is important because the information in the current data sets does not provide the data necessary to simulate the health effects of neighborhoods and segregation. Her group wants health data sets that are representative of metropolitan areas and have information about neighborhoods, because without them it is possible to lose track of the real issues that are shaping the unequal opportunity structures.

Dr. Bracho also had concerns regarding data collection. Her group, Latino Health Access, collects data from census tracts and from communities. She argues that these data need to be revised for public health environments, so that health disparities affecting young communities, which may not be evident in life expectancy data, can be identified with data that use smaller numbers of cases as the unit of analysis. There is a need for local comparisons to evaluate school performance, public safety, and environmental indicators such as open space on various concentrations of disparities. Those are the data that are useful to advance interventions.

Statistics do not always give a clear indication of what is really happening, continued Dr. Bracho. If someone analyzed the statistics for Orange County, California, for example, they would find that the life expectancy for Hispanics would seem quite high since it is a very young community. Yet the disparities are there if you know where to look. According to the census tract, only 3 percent of the senior citizens in the county do not have health insurance. If you segment the population and look specifically at Hispanics, however, you would find that 56 percent of Hispanic elders do not have health insurance.

Collaborations and Community Innovation

It is important to recognize that many of these problems involve more than one sector, stressed Dr. Acevedo-Garcia. She works with the housing policy community and the public health community in metropolitan areas, but these groups rarely participate at the same meetings. Although there is a great deal of discussion about how difficult those collaborations are, she is aware of few incentives to collaborate with other groups or sectors to reduce disparities.

Any community innovation template should have at least eight minimum characteristics, said Mr. Dotson. It needs to be multidimensional rather than focused on one issue, and it must be accessible, affordable, and available. We need to think of local implementation and local control as part of that innovative template. The final two characteristics needed are constancy—Can the community in which we are trying to implement this innovation depend on the program being there at a certain period of time on a regular basis?—and sustainability.

Addressing Health Disparities in St. Louis

The St. Louis Health Department has been advocating for a coordinated comprehensive approach to reducing health disparities for nearly a decade, said workshop participant William Dotson. In the next few months, the city will release a report, *Public Health: Understanding Our Needs*, the third in a series of biennial reports. This series of reports provides community needs assessments examining 64 variables categorized by demographic and socioeconomic factors and issues related to access and equality, racial polarization, epidemics, environmental issues, and injury behavior related to mortality. People use this report to gain a deeper understanding of the challenges of reducing health disparities and as a guide for writing grants and advocating for new programs.

Another effort by the city of St. Louis was the Racial and Ethnic Approaches to Community Health (REACH) 2010 project, which sponsored a community program targeting heart disease prevention. Despite developing innovative programs, establishing strong community partnerships, and countless hours of planning and hard work, St. Louis was not awarded one of the demonstration projects. There was an effort to continue the program with support from local foundations and private entities, but adequate funding did not materialize. Ultimately the decision has to be made whether or not to continue a program at a lower funding level, knowing that the reduction in funding could ultimately compromise the integrity of the original effort. This is a very hard choice to make.

Over the past three years there have been some changes in the city of St. Louis. Life expectancy has gone up, mortality from HIV/AIDS has declined, and more women have taken advantage of first trimester care. There have been improvements, but they are small. St Louis has a long way to go in terms of organizing in order to increase the momentum toward reaching set goals. The challenge now is focused on providing, implementing, and creating momentum for solutions that will address health disparities.

A member of the audience representing the St. Louis Health Commission, an organization created with a mission of increasing access, improving health outcomes, and reducing health disparities within the public safety net system, shared some information from their recent reports examining issues that affect communities in the city of St. Louis. Among their findings, the commission found that primary care access in the public safety net system has increased by 13 percent in the past three to four years due to regional collaborative efforts, and there has been an 85 percent reduction in the time that people have to wait for specialty care.

REFERENCES

Acevedo-Garcia, D., N. McArdle, T. L. Osypuk, B. Lefkowitz, and B. K. Krimgold. 2007. *Children left behind: How metropolitan areas are failing America's children.* Diversity Report Number 1. Harvard School of Public Health, and Center for the Advancement of Health, January 2007. Boston, MA. http://diversitydata.sph.harvard.edu/children_left_behind_final_report.pdf (accessed July 11, 2007).

BRFSS (Behavioral Risk Factor Surveillance System). 2008. *About the BRFSS.* http://www.cdc.gov/brfss/about.htm (accessed March 19, 2008).

Brooks-Gunn, J., G. J. Duncan, and J. L. Aber. 1997. *Neighborhood poverty.* New York: Russell Sage Foundation.

IOM (Institute of Medicine). 2000. *From neurons to neighborhoods: The science of early childhood development.* Washington, DC: National Academy Press.

IOM. 2002. *Care without coverage: Too little, too late.* Washington, DC: The National Academies Press.

Murray, C. J. L., S. C. Kulkarni, C. Michaud, N. Tomijima, M. T. Bulzacchelli, T. J. Iandiorio, and M. Ezzati. 2006. Eight Americas: Investigating mortality disparities across races, counties, and race-counties in the United States. *PLOS Medicine* 3(9):1–12.

NCHS (National Center for Health Statistics). 2008. *National Health and Nutrition Examination Survey.* http://www.cdc.gov/nchs/data/factsheets/nhanes.pdf (accessed March 19, 2008).

WHO (World Health Organization). 2002. *The world health report 2002: Reducing risks, promoting healthy life.* Geneva, Switzerland: World Health Organization. http://www.who.int/whr/2002/en/whr02_en.pdf (accessed July 11, 2006).

3

Clinical and Community-Development Approaches to Reducing Disparities

In preparation for this workshop, Drs. Carol Horowitz and Edward Lawlor coauthored a paper synthesizing information about clinical and community-development approaches to reducing health disparities. Their paper, "Community Approaches to Addressing Health Disparities," assesses the implications for developing actionable strategies and describes the benefits of—and approaches to—integrating clinical and community-based approaches to impacting communities and reducing health disparities. This paper, which is included in Appendix D, was presented by Drs. Horowitz and Lawlor at the workshop, and the workshop presentation of their paper is summarized below.

DISPARATE APPROACHES TO ADDRESSING HEALTH DISPARITIES

There has not been enough progress toward reducing health disparities using standard accepted practices, explained Dr. Horowitz.[1] Typically, community approaches to health disparities are made through interventions or other efforts mediated through clinical or community settings (Figure 3-1). Disparities can be addressed in a clinical setting by addressing issues related to quality of care. Interventions such as these can include enhancing the assortment of services offered, ensuring that appropriate treatment options are available, training and providing competent staff, or determining whether the proper organizational and care structures exists. If quality-of-care issues are addressed, health care improves. If processes improve,

[1]This section is an edited transcript of Dr. Carol Horowitz's remarks at the workshop.

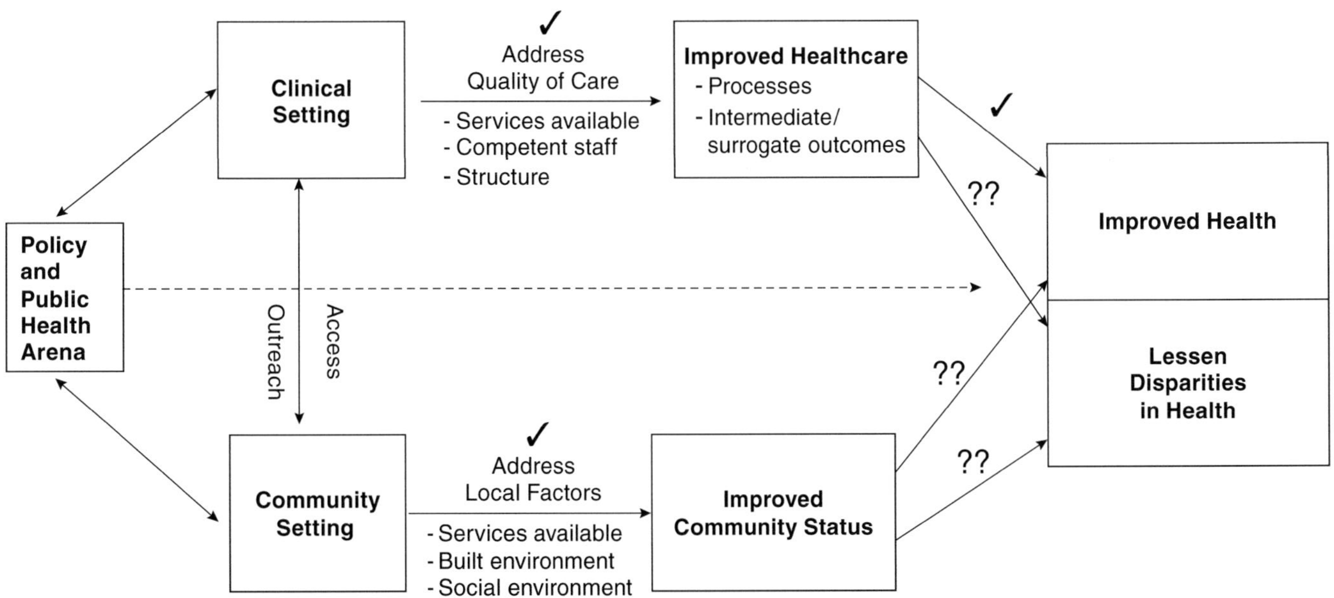

FIGURE 3-1 The "two paths" of community approaches to disparities.

some intermediate outcomes improve. However, although it is believed that improving health care and quality of care can lead to improved health, it is not always clear whether improving health care leads to the lessening of disparities in health.

The disconnect between health care and improved health in a clinical setting can be demonstrated by considering the relationship of breast cancer care and mortality rates. While there has been progress in decreasing disparities in breast cancer screening through mammography and disparities are narrowing in mammography rates, mortality rates attributed to breast cancer among nonwhites are increasing over those of white women. There are excellent treatments for early-stage breast cancer, but nonwhite women are less likely to get these treatments. In general, it appears that improving the processes—improving screenings and persuading women to receive health care—may not be enough to reduce mortality from breast cancer, especially among nonwhite women.

Similar problems are apparent when community approaches are used to try to reduce disparities. In a community setting, community building and development efforts address socioeconomic fundamentals and endeavor to enhance community assets. These efforts are varied but can include improving local services or the availability of affordable housing, enhancing the built or social environments, providing employment opportunities, alleviating safety concerns, increasing the availability and accessibility of convenient healthy food options, or ameliorating air quality concerns. Efforts such as these can improve community status, yet they may not improve health or reduce health disparities in a community. In addition, issues such as these can be considered outside of the purview of the primary program objectives; local factors are therefore not measured at baseline, making it impossible to determine whether or not interventions or programs effectively addressed these issues or impacted disparities in a community.

Silos

Efforts to reduce health disparities using either clinical or community approaches, but not the two approaches in combination, are thought of as silos. It is striking how many large-scale collaborative studies working toward the goal of decreasing disparities use a silo approach. However, programs that work toward reducing disparities using a silo approach can impede progress and potentially limit a program's success.

An example of a silo from a community-development perspective is the Local Initiative Support Corporation (LISC). LISC is a comprehensive community-development initiative working toward transforming distressed communities into healthy ones. In the last 10 years LISC has mobilized almost $8 billion to fund efforts to develop local leadership, create affordable housing, and stimulate commercial and job development in 300 rural and urban communities. Their website, however, does not define any specific health goals, and there are very few measures demonstrating health impacts in LISC communities. LISC is therefore a program that may or may not be improving health. It would seem that LISC could include health improvement as part of its programs, but that is not currently happening.

An example of silos with a clinical perspective can be seen by looking at diabetes prevention efforts. Nearly half of black and Hispanic children and nearly a quarter of white children born in this decade will have diabetes as adults unless something is done quickly to stop this trend. The Diabetes Prevention Program is a large, multisite national study that has demonstrated that if individuals can be identified as prediabetic—with sugars higher than normal, but not yet at the diabetes level—and they can lose weight through lifestyle change, diet, and exercise, diabetes can be prevented or delayed in a significant number of cases.

Interestingly, the study also showed that disparities could be eliminated in incident diabetes. Blacks and Hispanics usually have a higher incidence of diabetes than whites in America, but in the Diabetes Prevention Program, with the requisite lifestyle changes, there was no difference in the likelihood of developing diabetes. However, the study included only patients who came in for two full days of testing. Patients also had to keep a thorough food diary for two entire weeks and attend dozens of sessions at clinical sites. In the end, this turned out to be an efficacy trial, but the program did not really have roots. When the funding stopped, the results stopped. Without the Diabetes Prevention Program, people are really struggling with how to manage their diabetes-related health concerns, and, although the program demonstrated a potential solution for reducing diabetes, it is no longer being used.

East Harlem, a predominantly black and Hispanic, low-income neighborhood, is the epicenter of diabetes and obesity in New York City. In East Harlem, there are many different silos working on obesity. From the clinical perspective, doctors would refer people for surgery, give people medication for obesity, or refer patients to a nutritionist. Nutritionists were a scarce resource, however, and patients who were lucky enough to see a nutritionist found individuals who did not understand their culture and who would instruct them to eat foods that were unfamiliar, unavailable, or unaffordable. Yet the clinical groups were doing their job and were realizing some success but, on the whole, patients were still overweight and it was generally viewed as the patients' fault.

In the public health silo, public health professionals were developing and offering free exercise classes for the community. Yet the community members were not consulted about these classes ahead of time so they did not attend them. In the end, community members were still overweight, and the public health workers blamed them for not taking advantage of the free classes.

There is also the researchers' silo. The researchers were conducting programs like the Diabetes Prevention Program: well-planned, hospital-based, intensive weight loss programs. They received grants and published their results in well-respected journals. However, when funding for the programs ran out, the programs were not sustainable. In the end, people in the community were still overweight and were blamed for failing to continue the program.

Policy makers are in another silo. Policy makers established laudable physical activity standards for schools, so they were confident they had done their job effectively. All schools, including schools in East Harlem, had a policy in place that established physical education standards. However, a percentage of the schools could not implement the new policies because they did not have gyms. In this case, although there was a policy, people are still overweight and the community is blamed.

Even developers play a role in the silo approach. Developers were building new housing in the area, but they did not consider creating spaces for physical activity because it was not a priority. Neighborhoods therefore lack features like sidewalks, adequate lighting, safe transportation, and green space. The developers have done their job but the community members are still overweight.

A community organizer from East Harlem recently expressed her frustration with the silo approach, continued Dr. Horowitz. Over the years the community organizer has been courted by representatives from many of these different groups. She has attended meetings with them and she has written several letters of support for their programs and grants. Yet, when asked for her opinion about what is happening in her community, she says, "You know what? We are all still fat and sick." When she wants to try to solve problems in her community, she is unsure who to partner with. She does not know who will treat her as an equal and not judge her for being overweight. She is unsure who can help make an impact in her community, at the same time ensuring that her community is not exploited. She is unsure who she can trust to stop perpetuating a "helicopter approach" to research, in which people come into the community, conduct their program, and leave without truly making any community impact. The person coordinating the helicopter program seems to benefit from it, but the community does not. All of these problems demonstrate the problems with silos.

Pursuing a Hybrid Approach

A hybrid model combines aspects of both the clinical and community approaches to reducing health disparities. This model would empower and mobilize community resources and residents at the same time it implements clinically sound approaches to improving health. These programs could be focused on bringing the community into the clinic or bringing the clinical people out to the community. Challenges such as identifying problems in communities, finding appropriate solutions, conducting evaluations, disseminating findings, and sustaining programs could all be accomplished more successfully with this unified approach.

Dr. Horowitz explained that Jim Krieger, a member of the Roundtable, had provided her with an example of a hybrid approach when he described an organization in Seattle called Asthma Care. Asthma Care oversaw the construction of new low-income housing that was built using special paints and floorings to ensure that the housing was free of asthma triggers and therefore would provide a better home environment for people with asthma. At the same time, health educators taught people about how to care for their asthma and helped them get appropriate clinical care. Asthma Care demonstrates how a hybrid approach would operate.

A hybrid approach could also be effective in addressing issues of racism and segregation in a community, since community members would be welcomed as equal partners. This approach would provide an opportunity for health leaders to listen and learn from and with community members. Health leaders would have the opportunity to discover the power, wisdom, and ideas that minority groups in the community, or people directly affected by illnesses, have to offer. When the clinical and the community factions work together, there is the potential to transform power differentials and relationships and create opportunities for new ideas and new resources. The potential exists to create solutions that build on community assets, such as enhancing community partnerships; improving recruitment, retention, research, and programs; and successfully aligning resources with the most pressing needs and priorities in a community.

A comparison of the clinical, hybrid, and community approaches (Table 3-1) shows that clinical approaches do impact health, although it is unclear how substantially they impact health disparities outcomes. The advantage of the clinical approach is that it addresses biological determinants of health and enhances clinical resources and capacity. The disadvantages of this approach are that they have a narrow clinical perspective, the programs may be unsustainable, and it is unclear whether they have any residual effectiveness in the communities beyond the early trials that are conducted.

Community approaches address social determinants of health, and efforts may enhance both community resources and capacity. Some community models may also be more sustainable than others. The disadvantages of community approaches include difficulty in determining whether they are effectively reaching their goals, the long time lines that many

TABLE 3-1 Characteristics of Clinical, Hybrid, and Community Approaches

	Clinical	Hybrid	Community
Evidence of Health Impact	Positive on health, not evident in disparities	Emerging	Not a traditional goal, not measured
Advantages	• Address biological determinants of health • Enhance clinical resources and capacity	• Address biological and social determinants of health • Sustainable designs • Enhance community and clinical resources and capacity	• Address social determinants of health • Sustainable designs • Enhance community resources and capacity
Disadvantages	Narrow clinical perspective, ? sustainability, ? real world effectiveness	Challenging to scale up or replicate, time consuming, intensive to initiate	Target broad, time horizon long, not health specific

approaches have, and the fact that programs are not health-specific. In addition, because community approaches have not traditionally set benchmark goals, their impact is not always measured.

While the evidence is still emerging, hybrid models theoretically have the advantages of addressing both the biological and social determinants of health, the programs can be sustainable, and they can enhance resources in the community and clinical settings. The disadvantages are that they can be time-consuming, time-intensive to initiate, and challenging to scale up or replicate.

Community health workers represent an example of a hybrid approach that is clinically centered. These workers are often lay community members who work with the health system to help bring community members into the clinic. Often with similar ethnicity and life experiences as the patients, they can act as facilitators. Community health workers can help educate patients and help them navigate the medical system, as well as link patients to services or advocate for care. Involving community health workers can improve patients' access and help them decrease asthma symptoms or urgent care use or improve their blood pressure control.

An example of a hybrid approach that is research-centered is the general field of community-based participatory research (CBPR). This research involves equitably including the community as partners in research programs. All of the participants share power, funding, and resources. Although a young field, CBPR has uncovered some important barriers to care that had not been considered using traditional research methods. Asthma Care is an example of this approach, and there are other CBPR interventions in the areas of pesticide use and obesity, among others.

An example of a policy-centered hybrid approach is Racial and Ethnic Approaches to Community Health (REACH) 2010. This program is comprised of 40 separate projects that have been funded since 1999 with a goal of addressing disparities in priority health areas for certain racial and ethnic groups. REACH 2010 strives to ensure local leadership and community participation in programs that include prevention, education, and evaluation. Early results from the REACH communities versus controlled communities show that the REACH 2010 interventions have had some success with screening blacks and Hispanics for cholesterol. Some REACH communities have seen an increase in the number of American Indians taking blood pressure medications and a decrease in the number of Asian Americans who smoke. Although it must be stressed that this is a process that will take time, the REACH programs seem to be beneficial.

Challenges of Hybrid Approaches

There are several challenges to advancing hybrid approaches, including adapting the clinical enterprise, building effective partnerships, building support for empirical evaluation, and relying more heavily on public health ideals. There has been some progress in advancing hybrid approaches, but future efforts must move beyond translating materials into appropriate languages and cultural competency training. New interventions should maintain profiles of the communities they serve, collaborate with the community to meet standards for care, monitor the impact of what is being done to improve care in the community, and share how well the programs are reaching their goals. Throughout all of these steps, the community must be at the planning table.

Building effective partnerships is another challenge of advancing the hybrid approach. Who should communities work with? How does a community participate in a successful partnership? How can a community build trust with a potential partner? How do groups discover each other's strengths and work with them? How does a community cultivate expertise both within the community itself and across all the stakeholders? These are all questions that need to be researched and addressed.

There is also a need to build the base for empirical evaluation. It is important to understand the impact of the community development and community partnership approaches on decreasing health disparities. Large projects often have no health component and some smaller projects evaluate processes, but not all interventions evaluate outcomes. This is integral to advancing the hybrid approach and creating programs that can be replicated.

It will also be important to take advantage of public health. *The Future of Public Health* (IOM, 1988) describes the public health mission as generating organized community efforts, applying scientific and technical knowledge to prevent disease, and promoting health and affecting policy. We interpret this to mean that public health could be the conduit between these silos by focusing on health and discovering ways to prove whether certain environmental exposures or experiences impact health. However, to date public health has not had a role in leading integrated community-based efforts with a strong evaluative component. This void is a huge missed opportunity. There are also challenges related to solving problems of organization, financing, and policy that must be addressed.

Developing Hybrid Models—The Next Steps[2]

To advance a hybrid approach, it is important to understand the different issues that have impeded the development of collaborations that work across community and community-development health lines, explained Dr. Lawlor. Hybrid models should integrate community voices, community participation, and community ownership into disparity initiatives. These models should not be strictly clinical but should also involve education, housing, employment, and other fundamental areas that are integral to the process of improving disparities. They should have the ability to maximize resources, leverage different institutional players at the community level, and have a realistic chance of producing the kinds of evaluations and impact analysis that will be necessary in terms of advancing advocacy and policy agendas, to really promote hybrid models as viable approaches.

The paper, "Community Approaches to Addressing Health Disparities" (see Appendix D), details how hybrid approaches have the potential to positively affect social determinants of health. These approaches can also mobilize the clinical enterprise, which has been the primary driving force of the disparities agenda. The challenge now is to determine how to knit together all these disparate organizations and stakeholders—community leaders, community-based organizations, health care providers, funding sources, the world of community economic development, academia and academic medical centers, the public health enterprise, policymakers, the delivery system—to work toward a common cause. It is a daunting task. There are conflicting political agendas, different groups vying for control, and categorical funding limitations, among other issues that correspond to

[2]This section is an edited transcript of Dr. Edward Lawlor's remarks at the workshop.

each of these different constituencies. In addition, there needs to be a realistic approach for taking into account issues like resources and time frames and trying to determine how to have a quantifiable impact on disparities.

When considering these issues, it is important to have an understanding of the relative magnitudes of money involved (Table 3-2). It is very striking to compare the different levels of funding that support various forms of community development and clinical and basic science initiatives versus programs in which community development and clinical services come together. Given the aspirations and goals for reducing disparities and the magnitude of the social and economic changes necessary to achieve that, the levels of available funding are very minimal.

The National Institutes of Health (NIH) Human Genome Research Institute is a $484 million entity, and it is growing fast. There are new initiatives coming out of the NIH called Clinical Translational Science Awards (CTSAs) that are now in the order of $100 million, but quickly ramping up to $500 million in the next five years or so. The entire budget of the Agency for Healthcare Research and Quality for work on costs, quality, and outcomes of health care is $261 million a year. In contrast, the REACH projects, in many ways the leader of this kind of hybrid approach, is a $34 million enterprise. Considering that reducing health disparities is a national initiative, with daunting social and economic challenges, this is a very small amount of money to devote to attaining this goal.

There are other community-development efforts as well. As discussed earlier, LISC is one of several community-development investment corporations in the United States, operating in many of the same communities of

TABLE 3-2 Continuum of Spending from Basic Research to Community Development

Basic Science	Translational Programs	Clinical Practice	Hybrid Approaches	Community settings
NIH Human Genome Project	Clinical Transitional Science Award	Agency for Healthcare Research and Quality (research on health care, quality, costs, and outcomes)	CDC REACH	Local Initiatives Support Corporation (LISC)—for community development
$484 million/year	$500 million/year anticipated	$261 million/year	$34 million/year	$1 billion/year

interest that are being considered here today. LISC distributes $1 billion a year via grants, loans, and investments for community development. Another example of this kind of funding can be seen by examining Bank of America's community-development portfolio. This big, local, nationally known community-development investment bank, recently announced a $750 billion, 10-year effort to improve communities and community development. These are enormous investments; however, there are also tremendous overlaps in the agendas of the health disparities movement, both nationally and locally in community development.

Pragmatic strategies must be developed to tackle challenges and vet existing structures, solutions, and models to effectively move the community agenda forward. To accomplish future goals, funding sources must be reconsidered, and accepted standard practices should include community members having an integral role in the decision-making processes and general community participation for community-improvement initiatives. There is a need to develop community models that have the prospect of influencing large population health indicators and models that can be replicated so that successful programs can be copied systematically across the nation.

Structures for organization, governance, and funding exist into which efforts to reduce health disparities could be embedded. Regional Health Commissions, although they may be identified by different names, are organizations of varying size with the potential to bring together financing, community participation, and governance to carry out data-driven disparities initiatives. The Regional Health Commission in St. Louis is a version of this. Another example of a Regional Health Authority at the community level is the West-Side Health Authority in Chicago. For nearly 20 years this organization has been addressing community health indicators identified by representatives from the community and has tackled housing and employment concerns. Collectively, Regional Health Commissions are structures by which financing, participation, governance, and partnerships can all be focused toward reaching a common goal.

It is important for banks and corporations that support community-development initiatives and the people who work on disparities issues to work together. There is a great deal of affinity between the agendas and goals of these different groups, and by combining resources and knowledge, much more could be accomplished. Collaborations such as these should be actively pursued.

A variety of university–community partnerships have had varying degrees of success throughout history, and there are some famous examples of university–community partnerships in education and urban economic development. Last year, the University of Chicago announced a $100 million initiative to improve urban schools on the south side of Chicago. Although the university is providing substantial funding, the program is designed so that the community, the public schools, and the university are all active participants in the planning process and are all working cooperatively to reach shared goals. If models could be developed that combined resources such as these to address health issues in communities, great progress could be made toward reducing health disparities.

It is interesting to consider how CBPR enterprises could leverage their success by combining several CBPRs' efforts from across the country to maximize their potential to reach community goals or by ensuring that their programs incorporate providers, provider networks, and other institutions in the community. There are also provider networks or systems around the country in which multiple health systems and health providers map to certain communities. Provider networks organizations operate collectively, sharing revenues and resources, but they also work together programmatically on health care concerns and other issues that affect population health conditions in a neighborhood. Many models could be adapted or modified for the purpose of creating hybrid approaches.

It is important to think differently about how to measure, articulate, and value the outcomes of community-level investments. These investments should produce some return on investment in terms of improving health. Jim Keckman, a Nobel Prize recipient, has studied the returns on investment that are realized through preschool education. He is now promoting these programs nationally and getting support from many of the presidential candidates. The necessity of universal preschool is not a moral or an ideological argument, but rather a straight economic argument of the most rigorous sort. Universal preschool generates an extraordinary rate of return for society in general. It is this kind of thinking that needs to drive new investments in health and efforts to reduce disparities.

Some current analyses, which have the character of a social return on investment, fully account for improvements in environment, health, and quality of life, among other things, and are similar to some of the discussion at this workshop on some of the traditional, narrow, cost-benefit, cost-effective analysis. There are even some very interesting and provocative articles now emerging in the disparities literature that make an economic case for some clinical and quality interventions. If programs move ahead with the kinds of collaborations that are being discussed here today, they will need to rely heavily on both new resources and new approaches to data. Many people believe there is very little capacity to share data, ideas, or technical assistance and support, for doing the kinds of community-based collaborations that are being discussed at this workshop. Like a cottage industry, there are several little fiefdoms of investigators and projects. It is very hard to discern from this array of programs which models are working, what lessons have been learned, who the right participants are, or what supports are required to conduct programs in any systematic way.

A data agenda is implied in the work being described at this workshop that is really concentrated at the community level. In order for robust, community-wide initiatives to be built and defended, there must be new community infrastructure and resources developed at the community level. Communities must bring together an array of social and economic data, rather than relying on standard epidemiology or health indicators alone. New strategies are needed for evaluating the health impact of community projects. It will be necessary to find ways to bring together very different traditional sources of data—racial, ethnic, and geographic—at a community level. For example, the National Health Plan Collaborative is bringing together data sets from providers, payers, and demographic and epidemiological data, for issues related to health care. This kind of structuring should be done at the community level, ideally combining social and economic components as well.

As mentioned earlier, one of the avenues with a great deal of energy and innovation is participatory research. Many of these research efforts have been largely driven out of universities and now are in the purview of investigators. We believe that more and more effort and support needs to go to the community portion of those kinds of collaborations. These programs should increase community capacity and influence through resources, funding, and training. As investments are made in researchers' and investigators' capacity to do this kind of work, the communities must participate as equal partners, and there should be investments in activities, training, and leadership development specifically for community members.

Current participatory research approaches are episodic. They come with finite funding, and they go away when the funding is depleted. Over time, this process tends to be destructive. Communities become cynical and develop disdain for the process, initiatives are built and not continued, faith is lost, and the ability to sustain and have positive outcomes is unattainable. There should be improvements in funding and reporting requirements through the development of frameworks for funding that encourage continuity of programs in the communities in which they are operating. Ideally, new models should be developed that integrate funding, data, community engagement, and evaluation. Participatory research projects should be promoted that have broader benefits for everyone involved, beyond the kind of research outputs and products previously described. There are ways, in fact, to organize projects in terms of reporting, training, and interactions with communities that maximize the potential for making lasting improvements.

It is also important to consider community involvement in clinical enterprises in which communities and clinical investigators work in shared arrangements. Some of the CTSAs coming out of NIH require bench to bedside care. Increasingly, as the CTSA initiative has evolved, this definition has been changed to include bench to bedside, to providers, to communities. There is, in fact, an entire community engagement part of this enterprise now. The potential opportunity exists for creating more of these kinds of community–clinic collaborations, although there is no guarantee that this is the way that these initiatives will evolve. Considerable effort is needed to ensure that communities maintain an active voice in these projects and that community priorities are reflected in subsequent programs. Assurances are also needed that there is not simply token involvement of communities in what is largely still a clinical enterprise. In additional, researchers should be required to report the community impact of their programs to funders, members of the public, and members of the impacted communities.

Conclusion

Place-based geographic ideas should be taken very seriously. The time has come to think in a very rigorous way about each place-based community and to develop a deep understanding of the social and economic determinants of health outcomes in it. Intensive partnerships should be developed with community institutions and leaders to think about how money should be allocated and how resources can be garnered from some creative sources. There must also be a plan for rigorously assessing whether measurable progress is being made toward addressing health outcomes in particular communities.

To reach health disparity goals, a very different commitment is needed to partnerships than has been characterized in many disparities initiatives to date. The set of potential partners for these community approaches should be considered in very broad and ambitious terms. Already faith-based initiatives have been involved in communities, schools, other community institutions, and in such programs as the REACH projects and other disparities programs. Yet there needs to be a much broader understanding of who the relevant players should be and specifically who should be developing community-level interventions.

Serious thought should be given to embedding health agendas into ongoing community-development initiatives. Some of these initiatives are gigantic, not just in resource terms, but also because they involve so many community leaders who devote enormous amounts of time toward satisfying these initiatives. Many community-development programs in the United States claim that they improve the health of myriad communities. However, there are very few, if any actual health indicators, goals, outcomes, or strategies associated with those large projects. There should be some serious reconsideration of existing community-development initiatives and institutions, since these well-financed organizations are in a position to dramatically affect some of the disparities seen in the United States today.

Some serious attention is needed to data at the place-based level—specifically, data aggregating different sources that are shared with residents. Those data should not just be academic, but a vehicle for ongoing dialogue and shared agenda with the residents themselves. Used in this way, data can be extremely powerful.

There are some relevant funders at this workshop who think about funding investments in health disparities in very different ways. As in other types of social policy and programs, many organizations have organized their public and private resources around particular bands of intervention: health, social development, community economic development, and the like. In order to truly see progress, there must be collective agreement and sharing of the resources across these realms to make these kinds of initiatives of scale succeed. Medicaid and public dollars must be considered in this equation, along with foundations not typically associated with disparities, such as the Ford Foundation and the MacArthur Foundation. A way must be found to combine all available expertise and funding sources so there can be a measurable impact at the community level.

For years, concluded Dr. Lawlor, I have dreamed that we could create the equivalent of an investment bank for health in which capital from some of the big community-development initiatives and the provider sector could be pooled, and methods could be developed to focus and marshal those resources on investments in communities, with the results measured and evaluated. If this were to happen, we would expand the potential of our good faith and goodwill to individual projects and have the potential to truly alleviate health disparities.

REACTION AND DISCUSSION[3]

Following the presentation by Drs. Horowitz and Lawlor, several Roundtable members, sponsors, and audience participants joined the discussion. This provided attendees with an opportunity to comment on what they had heard, share information about programs and issues about which they were familiar, and ask questions or express opinions. Several topics were discussed during this time, including leadership, funding, intermediaries, community workers, and community capacity.

[3]The following discussions were edited and organized around major themes to provide a more readable summary and to eliminate duplication of topics.

Leadership

Dr. Nelson observed that significant monetary and personal investments have been made thus far on community-development efforts and the importance of incorporating evidence-based practice has been emphasized, but he questioned the lack of emphasis on leadership skills or training. Traditional forms of leadership created at the institutional and community levels may not be sufficient to work on these problems. He maintained that some thought needs to be given about future investments in leadership and what programs focusing on leadership might look like.

Ms. Glover Blackwell countered that she believes that there is a great deal of wisdom about how to build leadership because this has been done for quite some time. The Kellogg Foundation has a long history of investing in leaders, particularly leaders of color. There are also many leadership programs in different cities, such as Leadership Atlanta and Leadership San Francisco, among others. There have been a series of academic scholars who have looked at leadership and tried to see the role that it can play, and a number of people from the civic and business worlds have spent time trying to understand the elements of leadership that are important for achieving goals and objectives. We are actually fortunate if we decide that we need a new generation of leaders, because there is a great body of knowledge about how this can be done, she said.

What is lacking is a commitment to invest in a new generation of leaders, cautioned Ms. Glover Blackwell. The problem is not one of knowing how to create leaders, but rather an absence of public will. We will not have the opportunity to build on the extraordinary diversity, the most important asset this country has, unless we figure out a way to maximize the potential that diversity brings and incorporate this into leadership at every level.

We need to figure out how to develop strategies that start at a young age, so young people are encouraged to become leaders. Individuals could start in the leadership pipeline in colleges and professional schools, but there should also be flexibility to allow for people to become leaders in parallel ways. We should encourage them and provide them with opportunities to gain more exposure to mentors or participate on commissions or other hands-on activities.

Funding

Dr. Wong asked for further clarification about Dr. Lawlor's assertion that a disproportionate amount of money for health care is being spent on bench research—stem cell research, the genome project—rather than community empowerment and equity programs, which are at the core of social and environmental determinants of health.

Dr. Lawlor agreed that the allocation of resources was the central issue, stressing that communities can mobilize goodwill and community leadership, but, ultimately, in order to truly address underlying social determinants of health, thought needs to be given to where resources are being utilized and the magnitude of the differences in spending priorities between research and community priorities. Resolving these issues would require a fundamental change in political policy, resulting in a more equitable allocation of available resources.

Not all attendees held this position. Ms. Glover Blackwell noted that when she saw Dr. Lawlor's diagram showing the distribution of funding, she had a different reaction. The issue is not truly about the availability of funding, but rather whether the money is being spent ineffectively, she said. LISC, for example, leverages billions of dollars for low-income housing, but we should think of all the private developers that build housing. Much of what they build is affordable, but the people about whom we are most concerned do not have any access to those homes. The same can be said for the whole area of youth development and all the money spent on development and after-school programs. It is too narrow to think that a program designated specifically for health disparities is the only program working on health disparities.

Dr. Lawlor added that available resources at the community level should be more transparent. In Chicago years ago, there was an accounting exercise before the transformation of public housing that looked at all the funding streams for such programs as child welfare, special education, and so forth. The findings were astonishing, but they were not presented in a way that helped to establish how the resources should ultimately be allocated. It is imperative that the community understands what resources are available and how they could be deployed to actually affect some of the health indicators that need to be addressed.

Dr. Levi commented that while participants are asking community groups to design programs that are sustainable, there is also an obligation on the part of the federal government and other funders to make sure that their funding streams are sustained as well. Community members must look for the multiple funding streams and learn to integrate those funding streams into something that creates a true community-wide approach. There has also been discussion about new leaders who think along these lines at the community and local level. Perhaps the federal government should create a new structure that makes it easier for people to make changes at the local level. There was a logical reason for why each of these little funding streams existed when they were created, but they do not make sense in practice. Perhaps there is a model to adopt whereby the system could be restructured to make it easier for people on the ground to take these multiple funding streams and make some sense out of them.

Dr. Lawlor acknowledged that it is difficult to change the existing bureaucracy, but suggested that the Roundtable could promote the idea of bringing together streams coming out of the Department of Housing and Urban Development, for example, and funnel the funds to the various areas of concern for disparities. Although difficult, this would be fundamental for change to occur. Many states, and in some cases, towns and municipalities, are thinking about making changes along these lines. Although the effort is unfunded, Massachusetts has included disparities issues and the necessity of organizing a disparities agenda as part of its State Health Reform initiative. Disparities are grouped separately, and the state is working to determine how to overcome the structural barriers so that financing will be available.

Ms. Glover Blackwell pointed out that there is not universal agreement about the wisdom of combining all of the funding streams for designated entities. At one point in time, people who are advocates for social justice were very happy to see the federal government fund programs and be very categorical and specific about how the funds were allocated at the local level. However, many blacks, Hispanics, and others did not benefit from these funds, learning that they could not trust their local or state government to provide resources to their communities. Now there has been a shift, and people who have come out of the poverty movement, including blacks and Hispanics, are now in positions of power. There is a great deal of wisdom about how to make more effective use of programs even if funding for these programs is categorical, if communities can be more creative. But it is important to remember the lessons of the past.

Dr. Lurie said that while she has been working on public health issues and visiting communities around the country, she has seen little agreement about what public health is or what it ought to do. Some communities are taking on projects simply because they have received a grant to work on a specific health issue, regardless of whether or not that issue is a priority in their community. Not all community leaders know what the pressing health issues are in their community; they may not be doing regular community assessments or may have only outdated data. They stay afloat by writing grants and working on whatever they can get money for, whether it targets a specific problem in their community or not. This issue about federal funding streams is extremely important, but there also needs to be a system of accountability at the state or local level. Several other speakers have talked about the need to demonstrate that programs are getting results, she said. It seems like that piece would have to come together with more flexibility and yet, we do not have any great data systems or process for demonstrating those results.

Part of the solution, Dr. Lawlor responded, would require better organization at the community and local levels. Organizations must produce adequate and appropriate data and carry on productive dialogues with the community, and then translate that knowledge into compelling, important, and effective interventions. That is why it is important to know what structures naturally exist in communities and cities that might be the repository for that kind of information, analysis, and source of community input.

Ms. Glover Blackwell countered that she does not think that the structure naturally exists in a community, but rather it has to be consciously created. She referred to it as a community-building intermediary, an organization in the community with the responsibility of gathering and interpreting community data so that there is a shared sense of what the challenges truly are. Community-building intermediaries must be cognizant of what is happening in other parts of the country or around the world to see what is making a difference, and this organization must work with leaders in the community to put policies in place that incorporate what is working elsewhere so they can adapt it for their community or situation.

Power is in the hands of those with the money, commented Dr. Rhee. The NIH budget is $26 billion, yet only $2.6 billion a year are spent on disparities, despite the fact that NIH has identified health disparities as one of its top three initiatives. That $2.6 billion can still have an impact if you consider how much a program like REACH 2010 has accomplished with only $34 million. Yet how much of that $2.6 billion really goes to communities? How much trust or risk is really given to the communities? Ultimately, where the money goes is where the control really lies. Fundamentally right now, control is not really in the community's hands.

Intermediaries

Jill Thompson from the Child and Family Health Coalition in St. Louis commented about the role of her organization as an intermediary. One of the challenges her organization faces is that traditional funding streams are from clinical settings conducting research or from the university setting, and intermediaries fall somewhere between these two entities. Despite the fact that intermediaries conduct effectual research and work, they are straining to remain funded. The hybrid model leaves out the intermediary, and she would argue that they should be added. What role should intermediaries play, and how should these organizations go about getting funded, when even foundations question the importance of intermediaries, since they are not touching people directly? The Missouri Foundation for Health was singled out by Ms. Thompson as one of the few funders that recognizes the importance of an intermediary and has been very generous to intermediaries in the St. Louis region.

The Specialist for Health Policy at the Missouri Foundation for Health responded. The grant for the Child and Family Health Coalition was a community assessment grant. The Missouri Foundation for Health has given community assessment grants to a number of intermediary organizations in the city and state that focused on such health concerns as HIV in the community or such issues as determining why people are not getting necessary care or monitoring whether children are receiving adequate health care.

The Missouri Foundation does not believe that an organization has to provide direct services to receive funding. In a way, the foundation translates information so that the community understands what is happening in the system. The Missouri Foundation also funds people who can translate information to the community, such as advocates, or provide rolling grants for advocacy. This is a part of their theory on change and promoting health in Missouri through working with direct services, but also supporting change through the gathering and dissemination of information.

Community Workers

Ms. Boyce commented that she does not like the idea of community health workers, although she has been in public health for 30 years. Community health workers used to be called outreach workers. Community workers have been relabeled, but there has not been a career path created for them. If we were really courageous about workforce issues, she said, we would look at these workers, because a disproportionate number of people from these communities are locked into these positions. If we can move them into professional positions, we would not have to rely so heavily on people on the community to do ancillary kinds of activities.

A member of the audience responded that it is important to make sure that the community has a voice in the decision-making process in clinical and funding settings. For example, if the community has a real voice in a health care setting and someone was trying to move peer educators into becoming community health workers, community members could veto the change. In that way, the change could be prevented or perhaps some of the people would change but not others. Independent voices must sound the alarm when things are going wrong, she continued. It is important to have the right people at the table when decisions are being made. The NIH staff needs to be trained so that they can be active reviewers by ensuring that the affected community has an active part in the grants that are awarded. There needs to be thought given to the needs of the community and recognition that community representatives must have decision-making ability for health-related issues.

Community Capacity

Ms. Kubisch works in the area of community development, community change, and community building and she commented about the importance of community capacity. In the convergence between race and poverty that happens at the place or the community level, community capacity has systematically been undermined during the last 50 years in poor urban and rural areas that are primarily communities of color. While it was interesting to hear about the amount of money that went into community development through LISC and other kinds of health care and investments of health, people should not leave here with the impression that there are all kinds of nascent community development capacity out there in poor communities, she cautioned. The $1 billion figure mentioned in Dr. Lawlor's presentation consists almost entirely of loans.

The Community Development Corporation actually was started in the mid-1900s, with a view towards comprehensive neighborhood revitalization similar to what is being talked about here today, she continued. It endeavored to cross the divide between physical, economic, social, and political revitalization of neighborhoods. However, over time, for political reasons and for funding reasons, it became a kind of low-income housing producer. So although such institutions are potentially sources of great community revitalization, they are not doing it.

Over the course of the last 20 years, some institutions in poor neighborhoods have become affordable housing producers. They are service providers and they have settlement houses. They are faith-based organizations that are trying desperately to integrate services, to integrate the funding streams, and to do more ambitious transformation of neighborhoods. These are the most underresourced, low-capacity institutions that there could possibly be, stressed Ms. Kubisch. They exist under grants that do not provide overhead. They work on a shoestring budget. They cannot do community data collection. They cannot do any of the things that we were talking about in terms of local intermediary work. Their efforts are not being led by data analysis about where their communities are. They cannot organize. They do not have money for community organizers to try to empower the community and make demands on the system. Before turning over to the communities the responsibility of doing the work that is being talked about here, we have to realize that a lot of capacity building has to be done.

It is wonderful to hear members of the health community say that this is the direction they would like to move in, continued Ms. Kubisch. The health community has massive resources. They are powerful institutions in the form of urban hospitals, and there is a great deal of money devoted to health initiatives. Can partnerships between the health community and community development be formed that value the importance of building the capacities to do the work cross-sectorially? Can the health community bring power, money, resources, and political pull to really help make this happen? Community groups know what the communities need, but they also need powerful sectors who understand that there is a double bottom line: a social bottom line and an economic bottom line. That value system is necessary to help community advocates do the work they have been trying to do for a long time. Community capacity is necessary at the organizational level in terms of being able to do the data analysis, community organizing, and advocacy that will allow these funding streams to be pulled together.

REFERENCE

IOM (Institute of Medicine). 1988. *The future of public health.* Washington, DC: National Academy Press.

4

Successful Clinical and Community-Development Strategies

The Racial and Ethnic Approaches to Community Health (REACH) 2010 and the Steps programs were presented by Drs. Horowitz and Lawlor as representative examples of a hybrid model that combines clinical and community approaches to community interventions. An important component of the workshop was hearing presentations from people who implement such interventions in their own communities. These individuals shared information about how their programs were initiated, how they have developed, what some of their challenges have been, and why and how they are experiencing positive results.

Two of the presenters represent programs supported by REACH 2010, a $34 million a year enterprise administered by the Centers for Disease Control and Prevention (CDC). The national REACH initiative is a unique effort to address racial and ethnic health disparities as part of the Healthy People 2010 initiative. Since the inception of the national REACH initiative, 40 communities across the country have been awarded REACH grants to develop plans for tackling a specific disease in their community and then carrying out the plan through community-wide initiatives with minimal input from CDC.

Ms. Charmaine Ruddock, the project director from Bronx Health REACH, and Dr. Janis E. Campbell, the principal investigator for the Oklahoma REACH 2010 Project, spoke about programs that are being implemented with REACH 2010 funding. Ms. Nancy Williams, acting lead for the Steps to a HealthierUS program, a 5-year initiative spearheaded by the CDC for community-level programs, presented information about that program. Ms. Mary McFadden, the program director for Steps to a

HealthierNY, and Ms. Lisa Pivec, the director of Cherokee Nation Health Services, presented information about programs that have been developed and implemented with combined funding from REACH 2010 and Steps.

BRONX HEALTH REACH[1]

Ms. Ruddick presented information about Bronx Health REACH, a program operating in the south Bronx area of New York City. The Bronx REACH community is predominately made up people of color and the residents are very poor; this area is one of the poorest congressional districts in the nation. By almost every health measure, the Bronx Health REACH community falls short in comparisons to other New York communities and when analyzed against national statistics. The death rate for blacks with diabetes in the southwest Bronx is twice that of those living in the rest of New York City. Black men are more likely to get prostate cancer, and the death rate in the southwest Bronx is 50 percent more than the rest of New York City. These are just a few examples of the health disparities in this area.

The Bronx area has had a troubled past. In the 1970s, it was an area devastated by poverty and crime, and residents were fleeing. There was inadequate or substandard health care, housing, and education, among myriad other societal, social, and economic problems. Many of the organizations that had previously located offices in this part of the city, such as the New York City Department of Health and the American Diabetes Association, closed their offices and relocated to other areas. It was not until the 1980s and 1990s, when the Institute for Urban Family Health established itself by building health centers in the Bronx, that things started to turn around for this community. In 1999, CDC announced their initiative to address racial and ethnic disparities by awarding grants through the REACH program to communities across the country. The new Bronx Health REACH took the next year to plan a program for their community and worked to have the Bronx become a REACH grantee.

A Year of Planning

During the initial planning year, Bronx Health REACH conducted a literature review and held a series of 10 focus groups to help create and mold the coalition action plan. Very early it was determined that the community initiative would focus specifically on diabetes care and prevention, and the project would benefit the entire community, not simply one racial group. Hispanic and black residents were actively recruited to participate in the focus groups to ensure that the results of the discussions would repre-

[1]This section is an edited transcript of Ms. Charmaine Ruddock's remarks at the workshop.

sent a broad cross-section of opinions. When the results of the focus group were tallied, participants had identified three major health concerns—stress, behavior, and a distrust of the health care system—that they believed contributed to their poor health outcomes. These health concerns became the focus of the Bronx Health REACH initiative.

According to the findings of the focus groups, stress was rampant in the community because of pressures exacerbated by living in a depressed socioeconomic area and a belief that racism was pervasive in the community. Individual health care behavior was targeted because residents believed they had inadequate resources and information and because health concerns had to compete with other basic needs, such as housing. The focus groups also showed that people had a deep distrust for the health care system in the Bronx. Participants expressed concerns about enduring disrespectful treatment from health care providers, complaining about a lack of two-way communication with their doctors, nurses, and other health care workers. Many of the participants in the focus groups felt helpless, believing that they were powerless to advocate for themselves or their families in the health care system.

Other interesting information was gleaned from the focus groups as well. It was discovered that there were clear differences between the attitudes and behaviors of men and women who participated in the focus groups. Men believed that they needed to show restraint when they dealt with people who they believed held positions of power. They thought a great deal about how other people would perceive their behavior, and this deterred or prevented them from advocating for themselves or others. Men in the focus groups did not want to cause any disturbances and preferred to have other people work to solve their problems, leaving them to get whatever came their way. The women, in contrast, took a more assertive approach. The focus groups also found that the people in their community believed that there was a significant difference in the care that they had access to when they were on public assistance—Medicaid, Child Health Plus, or Family Health Plus—compared with the care they received when they had private insurance.

When the community action plan was put together, there was a recognition that the initiative must address three distinct groups—community residents, health care providers, and advocates or leaders. For the residents, it was believed that if they were provided with the right health information, they would become more active participants in their own health care. They would regain the power to demand high-quality care for themselves and their families and mobilize their community into making positive changes. For health care providers, it was determined that they needed to become more aware of health disparities in general. During presentations to providers, they denied that health disparities existed and blamed ongoing problems on the poor health care system. Such interactions as these motivated program planners to add an educational component to the action plan to educate health providers about health disparities facts that were without dispute. Providers also needed to provide respectful and responsive care, offer culturally appropriate and sensitive care to their patients, and improve the quality of care for their diabetes patients. Finally, for advocates and leaders, there was a desire to mobilize and raise their awareness and knowledge about disparities with the hope that this information would motivate them to fight for public policy and regulation changes and advocate for new health care legislation.

Bronx Health REACH was less concerned about programs and more concerned about creating a movement. Many of the community leaders had been active participants in the Civil Rights Movement who fought for neighborhood reclamation in the 1970s and 1980s. Because these community leaders wanted to radically change the community's experience with health disparities, they motivated the coalition to seek widespread change rather than instituting individual programs. Only a movement could create the extent of change that the community desperately needed.

Moving Forward

The Bronx Health REACH initiative was announced with fanfare at an event featuring elected officials, pastors, congregational members, and over 700 community residents. The key objectives of the Bronx Health REACH initiative were to develop and implement model community programs; institute sustainable health improvements through policy, system, and institutional changes; develop a health policy agenda; and mobilize community residents around that agenda. The coalition also seeks to educate elected officials about the changes that need to be put in place to improve the health care system.

Since its inception, Bronx Health REACH has worked hard to develop trust in the community. They have formed partnerships with such organizations as the American Diabetes Association and the New York City Department of Health, two organizations that are now interested in reestablishing a Bronx presence. With the Institute for Urban Family Health leading their efforts, they have also formed partnerships between coalition members and other organizations to bring about change in the community. From a core group of five members, 40 coalition members now support Bronx Health REACH, and this group includes health care providers, public lawyers, after-school programs, advocate groups for diabetes, and researchers, among others. The Bronx Health REACH program has been both a nexus for change and a catalyst for change.

Initially the Bronx Health REACH initiative started with a small number of programs: starting diabetes education in the churches, creating an after-school nutrition program, and creating a small fitness program. The changes and programs that have developed in subsequent years have been the result of an ongoing community-based participatory approach. After the initial nutrition programs were started, community members expressed interest in expanding the initial program offerings and creating more opportunities to learn about nutrition. Feedback such as this has motivated program planners to constantly modify existing programs or implement new plans. A culinary initiative was started, a Fine, Fit and Fabulous nutrition and fitness initiative began, and Got Sugar, a campaign geared toward diabetes education, was implemented. Separately, local pastors kept pressure on the program planners to work for public policy advocacy initiatives.

In 2007, a new Youth and Nutrition Program began, and Bronx Health REACH participated in a national initiative called the 50 Million Pound Weight Loss Challenge. With funding provided by the National Institutes of Health, another new program called Health Disparities: Navigating the Health Care System Workshop Series, was started. There have also been a series of focus groups and surveys to determine how to best communicate health disparities concerns, how to recognize problems related to disparities when they were encountered, and how to motivate people to mobilize around health disparities issues and work for change.

This work has had an impact on local faith-based organizations. Pastors now routinely incorporate health messages into their weekly sermons. The pastor of the largest church in the Bronx established a Wellness Center after becoming convinced that the church needed to help address the risk factors for diabetes and provide church members with a constructive way to combat the disease. Many churches changed their culinary norms by finding new ways to make traditional dishes. In this way they could maintain the foods that held historical significance for community members but offer healthier options to parishioners. The churches have also included health advisories in the church bulletins.

The Bronx Health REACH initiative has motivated many of the churches to redefine their role in the community. Many churches now see health equality as a part of their Christian discipleship. Although pastors did not initially recognize helping church members to improve their health as part of their role as a community leader, there has now been a radical shift and several pastors have become spokespersons on health disparities, both inside and outside their pastoral work. Many pastors have accompanied Bronx Health REACH representatives when they have led delegations to speak with the state commissioner of health, the mayor, and the state attorney general's office to advocate for change. Two pastors wrote theologies of sickness and equality last year, as a way of encouraging their fellow pastors to think of health disparities as an issue they need to adopt.

There has been a great deal of progress with the nutritional programs that were created as part of the diabetes initiative. The programs have grown from modest programs to ambitious efforts to address the nutritional environment in the community. Bronx Health REACH has worked with schools and after-school programs, starting a restaurant outreach and bodega (small grocery store) outreach program. It has also worked with communities, supported agriculture initiatives, and started a public policy initiative to address obesity in the Bronx.

The efforts of the Bronx Health REACH initiative have had a significant impact. Last year, the New York City Public Schools adopted a low-fat or no-fat milk policy for all the schools in the system. Bronx Health REACH was instrumental in writing a nutrition and fitness policy for the schools in the district, which was adopted by the school's chancellor for implementation in all of New York City's elementary schools. They also collaborated with the Bronx District Public Health Office and the New York City Department of Health on a bodegas initiative to have them supply more low-fat or no-fat milk. Bronx Health REACH has also recruited 11 restaurants in the Bronx to highlight their healthy menu options.

The Bronx Health REACH program has identified and established a seven-point advocacy agenda for public policy in the health care system. The first item on the agenda is to end discrimination in health care facilities, which was based on research on access to care, particularly for specialty organizations. From this research, a monograph called *Separate and Unequal: Medical Apartheid in New York City* was developed and published in 2005. This monograph had a significant impact on subsequent changes in health care provided by local hospitals. One local hospital, which initially sent out a press release refuting many of the concerns raised in the monograph, recently announced that it had addressed many of the issues raised in it. There has been extensive public education outreach and advocacy, and a video has been produced featuring individuals from the community talking about their experiences with health disparity.

Several lessons have been learned over the years through these programs. The most important has been to establish relationships with the right partners and to work hard to cultivate and maintain those partnerships over time. There is a recognition that for effective solutions to be recognized and implemented, they must be planned and initiated using a community-based participatory approach. Finally, if community members are provided with information and motivated to raise their awareness, they can take ownership and mobilize to improve, to reduce, and, hopefully one day, to eliminate health disparities in their communities.

OKLAHOMA REACH 2010[2]

When you give community members the opportunity to find solutions for their own community's problems, it is amazing what they come up with, remarked Dr. Campbell, the principal investigator of the Oklahoma REACH 2010 Native American project. The president's goal is to eliminate health disparities experienced by racial and ethnic minority populations in key areas by 2010. REACH 2010 demonstration projects, such as Oklahoma REACH 2010, are community-driven to mobilize and organize resources, with the goal of creating effective and sustainable programs and eliminating health disparities of racial and ethnic minorities, one community at a time. Oklahoma REACH 2010 will receive funding for only a few more months; therefore the immediate focus has been to create effective, sustainable programs. The community has been remarkably effective in accomplishing this goal and starting to work toward eliminating health disparities, Dr. Campbell noted.

Oklahoma REACH 2010, one of the original REACH grantees, was originally funded in 1999. Oklahoma REACH 2010 is a coalition made up of the Absentee–Shawnee and Cheyenne–Arapaho Tribes, the Cherokee, Chickasaw, Choctaw, Pawnee, and Seminole Nations, the Indian Health Care Resource Center in Tulsa, the Oklahoma State Department of Health, and the Wichita and affiliated tribes. The coalition is focused on reducing health disparities in cardiovascular disease, diabetes, and any associated risk factors through increased availability and promotion of physical activity at a community level. There was confidence that this goal would be supported by community members, and it could serve as a catalyst for other efforts.

Oklahoma has several REACH 2010 communities and the second largest American Indian population in the United States. The REACH projects cover about 75 percent of Oklahoma's American Indian population, although of the 39 federally recognized tribes in the state, only 8 are part of the program. There is a great deal of work yet to be done in Oklahoma. The Oklahoma REACH 2010 project was one of only two projects focusing on American Indians out of 42 grantees originally awarded Phase II funding. There are five American Indian grantees in the core capacity, meaning that their programs are funded at a significantly lower level than the other projects receiving funding.

---

[2]This section is an edited transcript of Dr. Janis Campbell's remarks at the workshop.

Tenets and Planning

The first few years of the Oklahoma REACH 2010 project were very challenging for all of the coalition partners, but it was during this time that a set of tenets and principles was developed to guide the coalition's efforts. These tenets include maintaining community control, equal responsibility and equal benefits, shared data, and tribal sovereignty. The tenet of community control had a significant impact on how the funding for the Oklahoma REACH 2010 project was disbursed to the different community partners. Rather than having the money controlled by one entity, a distribution system was devised whereby CDC would send the funding to the Oklahoma State Department of Health, which, in turn, would distribute the funding directly to the participating communities through subcontracts. The 333 actively participating communities, guided by a set of common principles, maintained the right to hire, fire, make decisions, and control their projects. This community control, as well as the flexibility and trust established and maintained by CDC, have been integral to the success of the project.

Ensuring equal responsibility and equal benefits was a tenet adopted very early. Every tribe or nation would receive the same amount of funding for its programs regardless of size or membership, but they would also be expected share equally in the workload. This tenet had a very positive effect on the success of the program, since tribes and nations vary considerably in their size and there had been concern that programs would be dominated by the larger entities. All data are shared and cannot be presented or published without the Steering Committee's knowledge and consent. To date, project dissemination has included 67 national presentations, 3 international presentations, 3 peer-reviewed articles, a book chapter, and a report. Government-to-government relations and tribal sovereignty have also been integral to establishing how the Steering Committee and the programs work.

Successes

The Oklahoma REACH 2010 coalition has enjoyed many successes. The coalition has helped establish a shared vision and mission among all of the partners, and programs have been implemented in every participating community. For 8 years, this disparate coalition of tribes and nations has worked together collectively to reach common goals. This is a powerful testimonial to the confidence they put in this project. Every participating community has started a new physical activity program or expanded an existing one and several communities have created programs with objectives that move beyond the initial goal of increasing physical activity. Although physical activity remains the primary focus, programs have been developed that focus on nutrition, education, secondary prevention activities, tobacco prevention, and health screenings through Indian Health Service or Tribal Health Services.

Staffing and infrastructure have been established, and approximately 25 full- and part-time tribal staff members have been hired in the community, although many are only partially funded. Nearly 75 community tribal members have been trained to lead different physical activity programs, and approximately 200 certified training sessions have been held for American Indian community members. Community involvement and participation have been phenomenal.

Community partnerships have been a huge part of the success of REACH 2010. Initially, each community partner received approximately $90,000 in seed money to develop new programs. Over time, however, many coalition partners have developed partnerships with other groups in order to pool resources and strengthen their programs. One example of this can be seen with the Cheyenne–Arapaho Tribe, a fairly large tribe consisting of about 12,000 members spread out over more than 10 counties in western Oklahoma. By demonstrating the success of their physical activity programs, they were able to convince the Gaming Commission of the Cheyenne–Arapaho Tribe to allocate 7 percent of the gaming funds to their programs, a contribution amounting to over $1 million a year. Without the seed money provided through the Oklahoma REACH 2010 program to develop and implement the pilot program, the partnership with the Gaming Commission would never have taken place. Other partnerships have been forged with local colleges to create health and physical education programs and with the Indian (or Tribal) Health Service, one of the largest partners in almost every tribe, which provides community health representatives, wellness centers, and health promotion and diabetes programs. Schools, firefighters, police, and local fitness gyms have also been partners throughout the life of the program.

The Oklahoma REACH 2010 project has an enormous number of exercise activities. Each week there are at least 75 activities and there are over 1,000 recreational events each year. Over 5,000 community members have participated in programs, 3,000 of whom are current, active participants who turn in logs documenting their progress. All of the programs have started, expanded, or enhanced a physical activity program in their area.

Since the REACH 2010 project began, tribal funding for environmental changes has become a priority. Wellness centers and exercise trails have been built, and walks and runs have been organized. Before starting the REACH programs, the Chickasaw Nation did not have any runs in the area; they now have four to five each year. These runs are extremely important because they motivate people to train over a longer period of time and because they are huge social events for the communities. Hominy, a small town in southeastern Oklahoma, hosted a Big Foot Run, which attracted 275 runners to the town.

There have also been policy shifts over the years. Some have been minor, such as switching from sugary drinks at meetings to water or Diet Coke. Others policy shifts have been more far-reaching, including the implementation of more than 30 ambitious policies that affect the availability of healthy food choices in the tribe area, changes related to smoking and exercise, and environmental changes. These changes have been challenging to achieve but have been effective for stimulating community change.

There have been many changes in the Oklahoma REACH 2010 community since the program began eight years ago. Although obesity has not decreased overall, the number of individuals who are getting obese has been decreasing. Disparities have been reduced, especially in terms of physical activity. American Indians in Oklahoma are now just as likely to be physically active as the rest of the population. Successful fundraising has taken place through such programs as the Cheyenne–Arapaho partnership mentioned previously and through programs started by the Cherokee Nation, a group that receives substantial support for programs started under the REACH project. The Indian Health Care Resource Center of Tulsa solicited support from foundations and other sources. It now has about $1.5 million in funding that was not available before the REACH program began. And a small tribe, made up of 2,500 members in Anadarko, has created a sustainable program by obtaining funding from a local university and other tribes to ensure that all of its programs will continue even if REACH funding does not. If the Oklahoma REACH 2010 project ends in two months, those programs will continue. It is ongoing efforts such as that will have long-lasting effects on these local communities.

Lessons Learned

Several lessons have been learned from the Oklahoma REACH 2010 initiative. Most importantly, people should understand that native communities can successfully implement programs. When communities are developing new programs, training and networking are critical. As a result of the REACH community training efforts, there are now physical activity specialists who are experts in the REACH communities. Communities must also control their own programs if they are going to be sustainable. Finally, maintaining trust between the project coordinators or sponsors and community members is critical. Researchers or people who implement programs must be trustworthy, and they must also trust the community.

One of the reasons the Oklahoma REACH programs have been successful is because the methods for implementation throughout the program have remained extremely flexible. The programs offered to community members have included dance classes, dances, karate lessons, weight loss classes, ballet classes, and an obesity camp. The program organizers were willing to try any program that community members wanted to try, and many of them were tremendously successful. In addition, trust and accountability were established with the communities, and there was recognition and acceptance that success is not always what is initially planned. Programs that community planners never thought would catch on have become very successful and are now sustainable in the communities.

This initiative has truly had an impact on the lives of community members. One community member, the Assistant Program Manager and Chair of the REACH 2010 Steering Committee, lost 90 pounds and is getting ready to star in a new DVD featuring three levels of chair exercises. She came into the REACH program with high blood pressure and diabetes, but now she no longer has to take high blood pressure medication and her diabetes is under control. She did not join the program for physical activity, yet she is one of the reasons that the program is successful. She was motivated when she joined and she is able to motivate the people in her community. Everybody in the community knows her because she has been such a driving force behind this initiative. It is people like her who best demonstrate how this program can make lasting change. The exercise DVD was developed with the help of the Creighton Nation, which is not one of the REACH partners, and it will be provided free-of-charge to any tribal member in the state of Oklahoma.

There are many new and exciting programs that the coalition would like to pursue in the years to come. There is interest in having the new physical activity training programs adopted by other tribes and nations in Oklahoma and also in having the programs implemented statewide. There is interest in taking the Oklahoma REACH model and applying it to other health initiatives, such as nutrition education or tobacco cessation training, among others. Another project coordinated by a local university, called the Community Networks Project, has been initiated to work with tribes and historically black towns in Oklahoma. There is a great deal of work yet to be done.

STEPS TO A HEALTHIERUS[3]

The Steps program is a 5-year initiative originated by CDC; requests for funding opportunities were accepted in 2003 and 2004, explained Ms. Nancy Williams. The fundamental goal of the Steps program is to channel money into community-level, rather than state-level, programs. Program funding goes to the state initially, but then 75 percent of the

[3]This section is an edited transcript of Ms. Nancy Williams's remarks at the workshop.

funds are redistributed to state-coordinated small cities and rural regions or counties. The Steps program also funds large cities, urban intervention areas, and tribal entities like the Cherokee Steps and the Cherokee Nation. In all, 40 communities throughout the United States were awarded Steps to a HealthierUS programs.

During application development, states, large cities, and tribes applying for the program were required to put together a community coalition engaging a wide variety of community partners, develop plans for leveraging funds, and have an actionable plan prepared to start a program. Applicants were required to plan evidence-based interventions using community and clinical guides and other tools developed at CDC or by other national partners. The proposed programs could not duplicate existing services, but they could expand the reach of an existing service or expand community outreach. The programs had to identify a specific target area and design an intervention that would directly affect the subset of community members within the target area who carried the most chronic disease burden. The programs also had to be evaluated locally and nationally. The Steps programs are required to work across three diseases (asthma, diabetes, and obesity) and three risk factor areas (physical activity, poor nutrition, and smoking), and programs have to integrate four sectors: community, schools, worksite, and health care.

One Steps to a HealthierUS program was awarded to Seattle–King County, Washington. The Seattle–King County program coordinators have worked very hard to provide integrated, coordinated health care to community members by developing a program that combines the clinical and community perspectives into a hybrid approach. They have case management programs that help identify individuals who lack a medical care provider and help direct those people to places where they can receive appropriate health care. They have community health workers with access to community resources who help match individuals to appropriate diabetes education or physical activity programs. They have also been able to obtain Medicaid funding for some of their community wellness advocates who work with asthmatics and diabetics. The Steps program in Seattle–King County worked to develop very broad-based partnerships. They work with the REACH 2010 program in Seattle–King County and with their local Prevention Research Centers, two hospitals in the area, and a large range of community organizations.

Other effective programs are Steps to a Healthier DeKalb in Georgia and the Boston Steps program. Steps to a Healthier DeKalb has focused on ensuring healthy communities in which community members live, work, play, receive education, worship, and receive health care. They have worked in specific neighborhoods and in the southern part of DeKalb County. They have also reached out to other community partners or coalitions, such as Morehouse School of Medicine and Emory University, and have very effective partnerships with Kaiser Permanente, the YMCA, and Children's Health Care of Atlanta. Steps to a Healthier Boston had a neighborhood walk and set up 51 walking groups in 7 target neighborhoods—Dorchester, Hydepark, Jamaica Plain, Mattapan, Roxbury, South Boston, and South End/Chinatown. This was one small program out of many they have done.

A Steps to a HealthierUS program in Arizona works in the border region: Cochise County, the federally qualified health care center in Nogales, Yuma County, the Cooperative Extension Services, and the Tona–Ogden Nation. This group has been working on both sides of the U.S.–Mexico border to reach people in adjacent communities who routinely travel across the border and because the tribe has members in both Mexico and the United States. This program has played a very active role in empowering community members to take more active roles in the community-development process.

From a national perspective, all of the Steps communities are encouraged to move toward policy, organizational system, and environmental change. These goals are not easy in the public health arena, but they are necessary for creating sustainable programs. Many of the Steps programs have been heavily involved in worksite wellness initiatives for large and small businesses. Emphasis has been placed on making changes to local school policies by creating school wellness plans or making vending machine policy changes. School health coordinators have been instrumental in developing and implementing wellness policies in the school districts and throughout the Steps communities. Steps programs have also been instrumental in instituting changes in the built environment, improving disease registries, and increasing access to quality health care.

The Steps programs have worked hard to establish national partnerships. The YMCA was a national partner and provided $500,000 a year for 4 years. This collaboration allowed Steps communities to work very closely with their local YMCAs to make substantial changes in communities. Through such partnerships as these, the Steps programs have been able to build capacity within the Steps communities.

Steps programs have advanced chronic disease control and prevention in 40 regions across the country, but there is much more work to be done. In the future, Steps communities must work more closely with community development organizations, and program coordinators will be encouraged to start disseminating some of the lessons they have learned to other communities that are implementing new programs. There are always lessons to learn and opportunities for improving existing programs.

STEPS IN BROOME COUNTY[4]

The Steps program in Broome County is one of four Steps communities in New York State coordinated by the New York State Department of Health, explained Ms. Mary McFadden. Combined, the four Steps communities serve about 700,000 New York State residents. Broome County is a rural residential county in New York, about 10 miles north of the Pennsylvania border. The population of Broome County is close to 200,000 people, and residents are predominantly white (92 percent) and black (4.1 percent). Roughly 12.8 percent of Broome County's residents fall below the federal poverty line. In some of the rural school districts, 70 percent of the schoolchildren receive free or reduced priced lunches.

Steps in Broome County has developed a hybrid approach to helping reduce health disparities by creating science-based programs that lead to sustainable policy, environmental, or system changes. The program specifically targets blacks, children and young adults; seniors; veterans; and rural, low-income, and disabled residents. By developing broad-based programs that build on the strength of existing community infrastructure, Steps in Broome County has created new programs that have enhanced benefits and features for community members. The Steps program builds capacity for sustaining successful interventions across each of the sectors and in the priority populations, working hard to weave its programs and public health agenda into the fabric of the community. It does all of this, however, while being severely underfunded. Four years into a 5-year grant, Steps of Broome County is eager to show the impact of their program and to show how much has been achieved with limited funding.

An integrated approach is taken with the program, meaning that the project promotes partnerships, works to avoid duplication of efforts, maximizes resources, enhances coordination between systems, develops systematic identification of common problems and gaps and shares opportunities for addressing them, enables sharing of data and best practice, and changes the business-as-usual approach. The program currently has over 100 traditional and nontraditional partners and continues to work hard to have a presence in every facet of the community, including where people work, learn, play, pray, and use the health care system.

Ongoing evaluation is extremely important, and the Steps program uses the Behavioral and Risk Factors Surveillance Survey (BRFSS) and the Youth Risk Behavior Survey (YRBS), as well as local-level data, to track the community's progress. Both the BRFSS and YRBS are specific to Steps to a HealthierNY and are heavily emphasized as data sources for determining Steps progress. The school health index is used as a model to identify where the greatest needs are and where problems exist that need to be addressed.

---

[4]This section is an edited transcript of Ms. Mary McFadden's remarks at the workshop.

A fitness grant is being implemented that will provide baseline data, including body mass index (BMI) and a physical assessment, for approximately 30,000 children in elementary, middle, and high school. The program has also worked with each of the county's 12 school districts to implement wellness policies.

Several broad-based Broome County Steps interventions combine approaches from the community and health care sectors. A Farmer's Market has been instituted at Mets Stadium and the stadium gives free apples and grapes to children during Sunday baseball games. Other programs include Breathe Better in Broome which focuses on asthma educational programs; BC Walks, focusing on organized walking programs; BC Breastfeeds-Loving Support; Farm-to-You, a five-a-day fruit and vegetable program; Rock on Café, a community collaborative effort to provide healthier meals and food options in local schools; Young Lungs at Play; Loud and Local Community-wide Steps Campaign; Mission Meltaway; and community gardens that have been started throughout the area. The community has also instituted a policy stating that they will not contract with any company that will not change policies or systems or make environmental changes that serve to improve the health of the community. All new programs must also be sustainable.

Mission Meltaway is an evidenced-based program designed to promote a team approach to healthy eating and increased activity, while fostering sustainable changes through systems, policies, and the environment. Mission Meltaway is an 8-week healthy weight education program focusing on black participants who participate in faith-based communities. This program has been instituted at worksites; community organizations; schools; state, county, and municipal government offices; senior sites; first responder sites; and in health care system facilities. The program is led by community members, who, after receiving training about the program, become peer leaders for others in the community. In addition to running the program, community peer leaders are also responsible for recording and tracking participant's weight, blood pressure, BMI, and physical measurement on a weekly basis.

Each organization that partners with the Broome County Steps Mission Meltaway signs a memorandum of agreement stating that they will create policy systems and institute environmental changes related to physical activity and nutrition, so their employees and community members will have more opportunities to stay fit. With the support of teammates, participants from partner organizations lead healthier lifestyles by adopting healthier eating habits and exercising more. These efforts, in addition to other benefits, prevent and control the onset of diabetes and create sustainable changes to support healthy living throughout all the sectors in the community.

To date, there are over 100 participating Mission Meltaway sites in Broome County, and the New York State Diabetes Prevention and Control program and the New York State Healthy Heart worksite initiative have adopted this program as a community-based intervention strategy for reducing diabetes risk. In light of the program's success, other counties participating in the Healthy Living Partnership NYS Diabetes Prevention and Control Initiatives, as well as other NYS Steps communities and Steps communities throughout the nation, are considering adopting the Mission Meltaway program. Even the hardware chain store Lowe's, a nontraditional partner, has initiated the program at their national headquarters, and they are adding Mission Meltaway as a worksite wellness opportunity for employees throughout the entire Lowe's chain.

The Mission Meltaway program has had a tremendous impact on the health of participating community members. Before beginning the program, 83 percent of participants were classified as being obese or overweight and 68 percent were identified as being at risk. A majority of program participants reported needing to lose weight (98 percent), a portion of whom reported wanting to lose substantial weight (ranging up to 200 pounds). Participants reported joining Mission Meltaway to improve eating habits, increase their level of physical activity, or to take part for social reasons. It is a group-supported weight loss program, and many participants have found that the group support motivated them to stay with the program.

Mission Meltaway has been successful in reaching overweight and obese individuals, as well as those who are or have been at risk for diabetes. All areas of measurement have demonstrated statistically significant health improvements, providing strong evidence of the program's success. Among other results, participants reported an increase in their fruit and vegetable consumption by approximately a half-serving per day; consumption of fast food, bakery goods, fried foods, processed foods, candies, and chips declined significantly; mean weight decreased by 4.7 pounds per participant, with a total weight loss for the program of 4,429 pounds; waist sizes decreased by nearly 1.4 inches, with 547 inches lost in total; and 62 percent of participants decreased their BMI by at least 1 point. Through targeted physical activity and nutrition interventions such as Mission Meltaway, Broome County has taken positive steps to achieve a healthier New York State.

CHEROKEE NATION[5]

I was born and raised in Adair County, which is the most heavily populated native county in Oklahoma, and I have been with the Cherokee Nation

[5]This section is an edited transcript of Ms. Lisa Pivec's remarks at the workshop.

for 16 years, explained Ms. Lisa Pivec. Both of my grandparents were original enrollees of the Cherokee Tribe, and my great-grandparents came across the country during the forcible removal of native Indians from Georgia, North Carolina, and Tennessee. I am very proud to be a member of the Cherokee Nation, and I am very proud to work for my tribe.

When I first started working with the Cherokee Nation as a Health Educator, I promoted women's breast health by traveling to small communities to talk about self-breast examinations. Although I believed that this issue was very important, I quickly discovered as I went into the different communities that breast health was the last thing on women's minds. The women I spoke to were struggling with more pressing concerns, like getting food for their children, trying to take care of their family, trying to keep the electricity from being shut off, or trying to make sure they had a home in which to live. Self-breast examination, although important, was one of the least important things that these people were trying to cope with. This got me thinking about how issues are prioritized in the community and how to promote healthy communities.

The Healthy Nation Program was started in 1994, through a grant from the Robert Wood Johnson Foundation. The original funding was provided to address substance abuse in communities using new approaches that focused on community-level interventions. Since substance abuse is systemic with other problems in the communities, early efforts began by having an open dialogue with community members about this issue. As members of the community ourselves, we realized that it was vital to get input from other community members if we hoped to create a program that would truly have an impact.

The programs that the Healthy Nation Program initiates benefit the entire community. All of the community health programs are open to tribal members as well as members of the larger community. The mission statement is that the Healthy Nation Program promotes healthy communities through increasing physical activity, improving nutrition, and preventing tobacco abuse. The priorities of the tribes are preserving the native language, ensuring that there are jobs and economic opportunities for tribal members in local areas, and investing in communities and community infrastructure. These priorities go hand in hand with the Healthy Nation Program efforts in the area of health promotion. There are over 100 Cherokee communities in the tribe, and this program works with approximately 30 of them. The work that is currently being done is centered primarily in five counties in eastern Oklahoma.

The Healthy Nation Program uses an integrated approach to address problems in the community (Table 4-1). Using the integrated approach, different programs are coordinated in a variety of settings, including schools, worksites, communities, and health care sites. Many health educators work

TABLE 4-1 Integrated Approach

School-Based:	**Worksite:**
School Health Index	Worksite Wellness Index
School Health Inventory	Smoking Cessation
Wings 4 Youth	Facilitator Training
Fitness Camps	
S.W.A.T.	
Community-Based:	**Health Care:**
Wings Fitness	Smoking Cessation
Community Physical Activity Events	Facilitator Training
Healthy Restaurants	OK Quit Line Provider Referral Program
Healthy Women	
BMI Screenings	

on programs that focus on a variety of disease conditions and risk factors, including diabetes, asthma, obesity, physical activity, nutrition, and tobacco use, in all four of the community settings. The Healthy Nation Program is a REACH 2010 and a Steps to a Healthier Cherokee Nation site—one of only three tribes funded nationally as a Steps site. The Steps program was originally funded in 2004 with a 5-year Steps cooperative agreement.

When planning a community program, it is important to remember that no single intervention will work for every participant. Programs should consist of various activities that appeal to a wide range of interests and skill levels, offering opportunities for participants to gain exposure to new opportunities and glean knowledge from their experiences over an extended period of time. When working with communities, it is important to recognize the relationship between people and their social networks and to respect that lifestyle choices are dependent on a complex mix of social and community environments. Community programs can either actively support or obstruct positive personal change. The Healthy Nation Program uses an integrated approach in order to saturate all levels of the social structure. Within the tribal entities, there is an effort to work closely with the community services programs, which oversee most of the housing and public works programs. The Healthy Nation Program also tries to work closely with the education department and the Department of Human Services. In this way, initiatives can saturate all levels of the social structure and institute programs that encompass and meet the needs of the community members.

One method for accomplishing the organizational goals of the Healthy Nation Program was to begin administering the BRFSS within the Cherokee Nation. Since 2005, the program has been able to oversample the counties and statistically analyze specific counties of interest. Using the BRFSS, it was determined that American Indians in the Cherokee Nation have higher rates of diabetes than other groups. In some of the Steps areas where physical activity programs were operating, it was discovered that although most people reported that they were getting the recommended amount of daily activity, American Indians in the Steps project area were significantly more likely to be obese than Oklahomans overall. The BRFSS also revealed that people in the Cherokee Nation reported that they were not consuming the recommended amount of fruits and vegetables and were more likely to smoke cigarettes.

In addition to the Cherokee Nation BRFSS, the Steps to a Healthier Cherokee Nation and the REACH programs incorporate many different planning and evaluation tools, including BMI assessment, weekly logs (database), referrals from health care providers, the Oklahoma State Health Policy Review, the School Health Inventory, OK Quit Line Data, the YRBS, and follow-up on smoking cessation programs. Another evaluation tool called the Knowledge, Attitudes, and Practice analyzes BRFSS information and tries to evaluate why people provide certain responses to questions. This tool evaluates how respondents' answers are affected by such concerns as lack of self-efficacy, skills competency, or the lack of infrastructure.

To improve the health status of the members of the Cherokee Nation, several new programs have been instituted. Programs have been started to coordinate and sponsor BMI screenings and direct summer youth and family fitness camps. The school health index has been used to help approximately 30 rural community schools develop improvement plans, which were implemented using tribal funds. Other programs include ongoing smoking cessation and tobacco abuse prevention programs and worksite wellness initiatives.

The Wings Club is an organization with over 1,500 active members that sponsors as many as 165 events each year. More importantly, this club has demonstrated how willing people are to participate in local programs when opportunities to do so are provided. If an activity is offered, there is an effort to ensure that it is accessible and that any transportation barriers are overcome. When programs are offered that people want, they attend and actively participate. In June 2007, a 5K road race was sponsored and, despite heavy rain on the day of the event, 293 people entered the race.

In addition to these programs, the Cherokee Nation has also sponsored hiking, bowling, swimming, Cherokee marbles, dances, and soccer in the communities. They sponsor any kind of activity that people might want to do. There are summer youth fitness camps, 2-week residential camps offered to fourth through sixth graders (ages 9–12), and day sessions are offered focusing on physical activity and nutrition. Day camps are operated in partnership with local school districts, so that camps can be implemented in communities. Evening sessions focused on skill building and traditional

Cherokee culture are also available. Family Fitness Camps are offered that emphasize Cherokee culture and incorporate healthy lifestyle tips and skills building. All of the camps are coordinated through local community organizations that are administered through the community services and education and human services divisions. A partnership with the Florida Atlantic University's Nursing Program provides nurses who complete internships in the Cherokee Nation as part of their master's program.

The School Health Index has been adapted and used to evaluate existing policies, make plans for improvement, and provide funding, technical assistance, and training to implement improvements at the local schools. Grant money and federal funds have been used in nontraditional ways, such as to build facilities and infrastructure, and purchase equipment. We also implemented a series of Tobacco Abuse Prevention programs. These efforts included funding the CDC Tribal Support Center, which offers smoking cessation and promotes the Oklahoma Quit Line; the Great American Smoke-Out; Students Working Against Tobacco; and 24/7 Policy Development, which has now been implemented in 14 schools.

In 2005, the Cherokee Nation began promoting the Oklahoma Tobacco Quit Line through local communities, providers, and the state of Oklahoma, translating cessation materials into Cherokee accompanied by Cherokee imagery. Of the 191 participants enrolled initially, 59 quit smoking—a quit rate of 31 percent, which is consistent with current research regarding quit rates. Of the remaining participants, 132 continue to smoke and 51 were interested in enrolling in another class. Since the initial program, the number of enrollees in the program and the number of people who have successfully quit has increased significantly. Other smoking cessation programs and the Tobacco Quit Line have also been successful. Disparity between nonnative and Native Americans smoking cigarettes daily is declining, call rates have gone up, and the percentage of American Indians who smoke is beginning to decline.

The Cherokee Nation has initiated a new program called Eat Better, Move More, which is focused on increasing physical activity, improving nutrition for elders, and providing nutrition centers. It is a 12-week program that includes functional testing and a variety of activities. Leaders from each participating group are identified and taught how to lead classes after the initial program ends. The program is being piloted at three sites and a manual is being created for systemwide distribution throughout the communities.

Program Challenges

The work that the Cherokee Nation does is very important, but it is just beginning. It has not reached its full potential for long-lasting change. The programs have been implemented and funded within the last 10 years, and it is going to take many more years to make lasting changes. There is a lack of physical infrastructure in the rural communities, and the rural service area is extremely large. There are currently 14 staff people who oversee programs in 100 local communities. That is why it is imperative to partner with other community services and education and human services programs. Local community members stated that they would like more individual exercise instruction, in-depth nutritional programs, additional group activities, and activities for special populations. Prioritizing policy adoption for health promotion programs in the Cherokee Nation has been challenging, as has strategizing implementation procedures and methods for reaching program goals and objectives. Recruiting staff and training individuals who are invested in their local community and willing to stay involved in the long term has been increasingly difficult, and managing competing priorities among program participants has been an ongoing challenge.

Looking Forward

Programs under development will be framed around curriculum-based group activities that provide social support from the local community to ensure that community members have an opportunity to participate in different activities at the local level and start developing new skills. There is a focus on sustainability using community strategies, mutual contribution, providing options for communities, and direct funding to provide community groups with the financial capital necessary to carry out community projects and learn how to manage the essential processes. Partnerships are being formed to help ensure the continuity of existing programs. Community-level interventions are getting under way and there are efforts to change health conditions at the local level.

5

Health Disparities in a Business Environment

Many approaches have been taken to addressing health disparities beyond the work that has been done through clinical or community interventions. Myriad organizations have developed successful strategies and programs to reduce health disparities using a variety of methods. By hearing from representatives of organizations making such efforts, the Roundtable members sought to learn about how specific programs have worked to reach their goals and what challenges or successes they have realized while trying to effect change among their constituencies. This chapter summarizes presentations by Ms. Diane Schwartz, the president of the American Conference on Diversity; Dr. Angela Glover Blackwell, the founder and Chief Executive Officer (CEO) of PolicyLink; and Ms. Katherine Gottlieb, the president and CEO of Southcentral Foundation.

AMERICAN CONFERENCE ON DIVERSITY[1]

The American Conference on Diversity is a nonprofit human relations organization in the New Jersey area that focuses on recognizing the value of diversity, educating leaders, and promoting respect while working on a broad spectrum of issues, explained Ms. Schwartz. The organization does not conduct clinical studies; rather, it informs the business community about issues regarding health disparities, as well as training and educating people about issues relating to diversity and inclusion. This organization acts as a

[1]This section is an edited transcript of Ms. Diane Schwartz's remarks at the workshop.

laboratory in many ways, working to achieve goals that few other organizations are attempting and seeks innovative methods for changing deep-rooted beliefs and institutional procedures that can affect health disparities.

A recent project focused on developing a Cultural Competency Training Program and educating trainers to administer the program in hospitals throughout New Jersey. After the program was initiated, the American Conference on Diversity developed an interest in extending awareness of health disparities to businesses that are headquartered in New Jersey. For most businesses, service provision, shareholder value, and operations are the primary focus. While benefits are provided equally to all employees, little attention has been paid to addressing issues related to the health disparities among them and the impact that these health disparities have on the company's performance. The American Conference on Diversity believes, however, that businesses should be aware that when their employees experience problems brought about by the health disparities they experience, these problems—such as increased sick time, absenteeism, and family leave costs—impact the bottom line.

Businesses must realize that there are real bottom line costs associated with health disparities, Schwartz commented. According to the Integrated Business Benefits Institute, the full cost of employee absences is more than four times the total medical payment; absence-related costs alone amount to 76 percent of net income when considering lost productivity from absence and wage replacement benefits. According to Schwartz, that is the awareness message that businesses need to take away from this information. In New Jersey, about a third of employees are members of racial and ethnic minorities, and those employees and their families are affected by health disparities regardless of their income or where they live. By reducing health disparities, businesses have a tremendous opportunity to positively impact their employees' health and quality of life, as well as the companies' bottom line.

What steps can the business community take to reduce disparities among their employees? Determining a means for reaching these goals is extremely challenging. Privacy issues severely limit how data can be gathered, and even such issues as determining which racial or ethnic group employees belong to are big stumbling blocks. Businesses would have to develop a method for tracking disease, before they could begin to determine the most effective ways to impact the health of their employees and their families. For more than a year, the American Conference on Diversity has been evaluating these issues and developing strategies for tackling some of these problems. Although we do not yet have all the solutions, Schwartz observed, we are closer to finding some answers and to developing processes for reducing health disparities in business settings.

To help address some of the challenges of reducing health disparities through business initiatives, the American Conference on Diversity convened a roundtable that included the medical directors of Prudential Financial and Horizon Mercy, a medical economist from Pfizer, a senior vice president from the New Jersey State Chamber of Commerce, and a physician who works in the area of cultural competency. As a result of those discussions, materials were developed to help explain to business leaders how health disparities impact a company's bottom line. It is imperative that businesses understand that, to be proactive about positively impacting health disparities and their own costs, internal changes in their own business environments can tremendously impact their employee's experiences.

Last June, as part of its Business Leaders Series, the American Conference on Diversity held a forum called the Health Disparities Score Card for all businesses across New Jersey, with the purpose of creating awareness and educating employers about health disparities issues. This forum included very disparate companies and organizations that were interested in these issues, including Johnson & Johnson, the American Association of Retired Persons, Newark Liberty International Airport, major national and regional employers, and local hospitals. The forum provided information and offered strategies for businesses to follow to benefit their employees, reduce costs, and reduce health disparities for themselves and their families.

At the forum, several of New Jersey's larger employers reported that they have engaged third parties to mine their data to collect information about their employees' health in general, so the employers can begin to develop their own internal programs. Many of these large, global companies have developed affinity groups, which mentor groups of employees who share race or ethnicity and help them advance their professional careers. As these employers begin to understand how health disparities affect their employees' experiences, they are starting to focus on specific wellness and health-related programs.

Moving Forward One Business at a Time

To date, the focus has been to spread the message about health disparities to larger companies, yet the American Conference on Diversity would like medium-size companies to know that they also have a stake in this issue. Regional outreach is being planned so working groups can be created to help the companies that care about these issues to make strategic changes. It is important for all employers to recognize that companies can prosper while providing for their employees' health-related needs. The American Conference on Diversity would also like to begin pushing for changes in the insurance industry. If large employers start asking their insurance providers to provide incentives in their plan offerings, employees may be more likely to adopt better health practices. Providing free mammograms or other routine tests, for example, could result in more employees receiving yearly screenings and other preventive care.

Although agreeing with Drs. Horowitz and Lawlor that clinical and community efforts can be combined to address the issue of health disparities, Schwartz observed that the business community can also review its current practices. Businesses focus on the bottom line, but there is a very real case to be made for making internal changes to affect the health of their workforce and, in turn, change their communities. Schwartz believes that insurers will soon start providing new programs and plans that address health disparities issues, and some larger insurers across the country either already have the data or are starting to gather them to address these issues. Change is coming, and the American Conference on Diversity is continuing to encourage the awareness that creates positive change.

Reaction and Discussion[2]

Dr. Lurie asked if there were any specific approaches or ways of framing the health disparities issues for the business community that have been more successful than others. Ms. Schwartz explained that she has found that the most compelling messages always come down to money and the bottom line for businesses. However, she believes that businesses should not just pay attention to health care costs; they should also direct their human resource staff to seriously delve into these issues to determine the impact of health disparities on their business in general. This is a very big step for some businesses to take. It has been difficult to convince companies to commit to changing their policies and pledging to compile and analyze their employees' health data and use that information to improve health care and benefits packages for their workforce.

Dr. Suggs agreed that businesses are primarily focused on making a profit. No matter what kind of business it is, it must be cognizant of the disproportionate health care costs it has to absorb in comparison to its competitors. Many businesses are looking at these issues in a more serious way for the first time. But when it comes to making changes in the existing arrangements, some people with powerful interests want things to remain as they are because they have been successful with the status quo. Still, there are compelling reasons why the status quo is not acceptable. Businesses can make a judgment based on their economic well-being and decide that they cannot afford to continue to absorb these kinds of health care costs—that it is truly time for a change.

Dr. Levi also agreed, adding that people need to be leading healthier

[2]The following discussions were edited and organized around major themes to provide a more readable summary and to eliminate duplication of topics.

lives. Employers should worry not only about the wellness of their current employees and their families, but also about the wellness of future employees. Future employees do not necessarily need a wellness program to make them healthy, but they need a program now to ensure that they will be healthy when they join the workforce.

POLICYLINK[3]

PolicyLink is a national organization staffed by a team of dedicated professionals, only a few of whom have experience working in the health community, explained Ms. Glover Blackwell. As a public interest lawyer, most of her work has been in the area of community building and community and policy development, and all of the people who work at PolicyLink have similar credentials. The organization is devoted to developing a new generation of policies to achieve economic and social equity in order to build a society in which everyone can participate and prosper.

When PolicyLink began its work, it focused on understanding the root causes of continuing inequality and inequity in America. Based on data, observation, and insight, Glover Blackwell explained, we concluded that where one lives in America has become an absolute proxy for opportunity. Where a person lives determines whether or not their children get to go to a good school or whether or not they live near good employment opportunities or have access to a transit system that enables them to travel to and from their job. Where one lives determines whether or not one's family will have access to money quickly if there is a crisis. People living in some communities can quickly pull money out of their homes because they are constantly increasing in value, whereas people living in other communities do not have similar opportunities or options.

The people at PolicyLink realized that where people live determines how healthy they are, how long they are going to live, and their general sense of well-being. Where people live determines whether or not they have access to fresh fruits and vegetables, whether or not they have access to safe streets where they can get out and walk around, whether or not they have access to parks and other places to get physical activity, whether the air is safe to breath in a neighborhood, or whether people live in a place where asthma is going to be a continuing problem.

Based on that insight, PolicyLink studied the work that people were doing in communities and began to tease out the implications for policy—local, state, and national—that could really build on this observation about the importance of place. We began to conduct research, train advocates, and support policy campaigns to try to make a difference, Glover Blackwell

[3]This section is an edited transcript of Ms. Glover Blackwell's remarks at the workshop.

noted. These efforts led us to start the PolicyLink Center for Health and Place, where we could bundle all the work we had been doing but also be more deliberate about identifying the next steps to take. We are involved in this work all over the country, from California to Washington, D.C., from the Mississippi delta to the Gulf region. What has been said here today suggests several things in terms of strategies.

She observed that Dr. Lawlor's discussion of the Local Initiative Support Corporation (LISC) suggests that it is important to join forces with other initiatives to influence them and to help them achieve the goals that are consistent with one's own insights. LISC is one of the biggest intermediaries doing community-development work in this country, and much of it, throughout the years, has focused on housing. During her presentation, Dr. Acevedo-Garcia pointed out the need for housing opportunities in communities that are rich with opportunity, yet LISC has spent $1 billion on housing in low-income communities with concentrated poverty. This is really the opposite of what Dr. Acevedo-Garcia was suggesting, noted Glover Blackwell. The reason for the LISC focus on communities with concentrated poverty is not because LISC does not understand how valuable it would be to live in communities rich with opportunity, but because all of the money it has been leveraging has been coming from low-income housing tax credits, a federal program that provides housing opportunity. One of the requirements for the low-income housing tax credits is that they can be used only in low-income communities. This is an opportunity for people who believe that where a person lives can impact opportunity to join with a vast network of people who have been doing housing and community development and would like to be able to see those investments happen in places that are rich with opportunity.

From developing strategies and conducting research, PolicyLink wants to find people who have a common interest in what we are trying to achieve and to join with them, Glover Blackwell noted. We believe that it is very important to get policies in place to put more affordable housing into suburban communities that have more opportunity. We have also found out that it is not enough just to have a policy that creates more rental housing and more affordable housing. With the nation's long legacy of race discrimination, for the most part, just putting that program in place will create more affordable housing opportunities for people who are white and understand how to make systems work for themselves. There is nothing wrong with that; we want more people who understand how to make systems work for themselves. Yet, for the new strategies to actually get to the disparities issue and to affect the people who are being left behind, we have to work with community-development corporations. Many such organizations are in the LISC network, so that they can work with the constituency to make sure they know about housing opportunities. They are getting people ready to move to new areas, and they are working in the new communities to make sure that they are welcoming and have the kinds of services and supports that people need in order to be successful. We need to find intermediaries that are working with large numbers of people and running these projects because they deal with real money and real government programs. We need to help them understand how their work improves the possibility of health and well-being for these individuals and families.

Additional effective programs need to be implemented. Receiving support from a government agency in the form of foundation grants or innovative programs encourages insight and learning. The earlier discussion about race is also very instructive. Many of the programs that are funded and are effective at helping people, whether they benefit Native Americans, Latinos, Asians, or very-low-income white people or blacks, generate enormous insight on how to work directly with community members to ensure that the communities' collective wisdom and preferences are truly reflected in the program structure. Too often, a successful program is started in a community but the money runs out, the leader moves on, the community changes, and the program is lost. It is essential to be very deliberate when initiating new programs to ensure that they are appropriate and sustainable.

Another insight at PolicyLink is how important it is to make sure that individuals in communities have access to fresh fruits and vegetables. It is terrible to blame people for not eating fruits and vegetables when they do not have access to them in their neighborhoods. Some fabulous programs around the country have been starting farmers' markets, helping local convenience stores successfully carry fresh fruits and vegetables, and getting full-service supermarkets in underserved communities. Insights such as these should be fused into programs that operate on a larger scale.

For example, the Fresh Food Financing Initiative in Pennsylvania has put close to $80 million into making sure that underserved communities have access to full-service grocery stores. With the help of organizations that know how to work in different communities, the initiative was able to finance the grocery stores and also learn what makes a program like this a success.

Focusing on leadership is another important intervention. There have been many examples in the Racial and Ethnic Approaches to Community Health (REACH) and Steps programs in which individual leaders have been essential in being able to inspire a community. They have been able to work with public officials to make sure that they are paying attention to the community. People have been able to transform communities because they understood how to translate from program and practice into policy. We need to concern ourselves with those segments of the community that are being left behind because of health disparities, and we need to make sure that individuals who are tied to these communities because of their history and their personal commitment, who are often members of racial or ethnic minorities, are identified, promoted, and supported as leaders, Glover Blackwell said.

Several of the previous presenters observed that they were not solely responsible for their program's success, but rather the program succeeded because they worked with dedicated, trusted leaders in the communities who were committed to the well-being of their community. It is not sufficient simply to advance a new generation of policies that build on the insight that where one lives impacts health and well-being. It is also important to advance a new generation of leaders, ones who can work at the community level and develop and advance policy work. Until we are able to move from addressing community needs and community insight to the world of policy, we will be forever working at the edges.

SOUTHCENTRAL FOUNDATION[4]

Ms. Gottlieb began by describing the state of Alaska as approximately 586,000 square miles that are home to 650,000 people, about 120,000 of whom are Alaskan Native people. In 1987, when she started working at Southcentral Foundation, it had a budget of $3 million and about 24 staff members. The Alaska Native Medical Center is a hospital with 150 beds, and she is the president and CEO of the Primary Services offered through the hospital.

She recounted personal details of her life, which have given her motivation to change the health care system in Alaska for as long as she can remember. She was born in the Kodiak Islands and is Alaskan Native and Filipino. The village where she grew up had approximately 100 people. She was 16 when she had her first child and is now the mother of 6 children. She finished high school with a GED. She grew up in a family of 12 with an alcoholic and a great deal of domestic violence and abuse in the home. Two of her siblings died at very early ages.

While working at Southcentral Foundation, she earned a bachelor's degree in organizational development and a master's degree in business. At the same time, changes were taking place in the health care system for Alaskan Natives, she recounted, as we assumed the role of managing our health care from the federal government and as customer-owners created a paradigm shift.

Southcentral Foundation has redefined the entire medical system for Alaskan Native and American Indian people living in Anchorage, the Mat-Su Valley, and 60 rural villages in the Anchorage Service Unit. There are now medical teams and primary care physicians in place. When people need care, they can visit the hospital and see their own provider on the

[4]This section is an edited transcript of Ms. Katherine Gottlieb's remarks at the workshop.

same day. In addition to their provider, each person has a medical team—a nurse case manager, a case management support person, certified medical assistants, a behavioral consultant, and a pharmacist. Gottlieb was involved in making the decisions about funding redesign and saying what she, as a customer-owner of the health care system, wanted to happen. Rather than creating more complexity, Southcentral developed a system that incorporates effective coaching, coordinating, teaching, modeling, and partnering directly with primary care physicians. It created a system in which patients work collaboratively with their physician to treat body, mind, and spirit—a system in which power is maintained by individuals and family members. Cultural competency is at the central core of everything it does and all services are added with this in mind, not the other way around.

Southcentral Foundation has enjoyed great success. Primary care patient visits to specialty clinics have dropped. Instead of seeing a specialist, patients are being cared for by their own primary care providers. Hospital visits per 1,000 primary care patients have dropped. Since Southcentral assumed management in 1997 and took control from the government, child immunization rates have increased and the number of hospitalizations attributable to asthma has declined.

Gottlieb observed that one of the most important messages she heard from the presentation by Drs. Lawlor and Horowitz about the hybrid approach involves having an effective leader. If the true leaders in a community get involved in making decisions and people in power listen to what they say, change can happen. There should also be shared responsibility. In her community, health care provisions are determined by people who are directly involved in the decision-making process. By taking control of their own health care, they have had an overwhelming impact on the community, and health statistics have dramatically improved.

By taking responsibility and ownership, she said, we have a say in what happens in our health care system. There is a shift in responsibility; it is now our own fault if something does not happen. We can not blame problems on anyone else. We also know if something is wrong, we can work to try to fix it. Although the resources of Southcentral Foundation are limited, she can influence the tribal entity to advocate for them to be applied to health care. A substantial portion of the funds generated are funneled right back into health care initiatives.

An initiative Southcentral has been working on is reducing tobacco use in Alaska. The entire community has become involved in this effort. Laws have been changed so that people can no longer smoke in public places, and the state of Alaska is working on raising taxes for cigarettes. Most public buildings and the entire hospital campus, including all of the off-site facilities, have gone smoke-free. We have worked very hard, she said, to educate people about the dangers of smoking, and we have developed a media campaign to advertise the fact that cancer attributed to smoking is the number one killer among Alaskan Natives and American Indians.

Gottlieb noted that several workshop discussions have focused on the value of creating partnerships with local churches and advocating with them as a community. Southcentral has attempted to do this, but with only limited success. One local church formed a nonprofit organization and is in direct competition with Southcentral for health care. Even as we were working with them, they were establishing mini-clinics around the state and drawing resources away from Southcentral. These clinics duplicate existing services and do not offer continuity of care. Other partnerships with local churches have been very successful. We have been working with one local church to help address issues of domestic violence and child abuse and neglect. This church has listened to our approaches for addressing these issues and has allocated resources toward our initiative to reduce domestic violence, child abuse, and child neglect.

The day's presentations, Gottlieb concluded, suggest that I should go back home and work harder to include the entire community of Alaska in our efforts. Our target population has been Alaskan Native and American Indians, but I would like to hear from the municipality, the government, and the other three hospitals in our area, about what they are doing to eliminate domestic violence and child abuse and neglect. I would like to know what they are doing to effect change around diabetes, obesity, asthma, and all the other health-related disparities in our state. There has been a great deal of mistrust among these different entities. In order for us to form a partnership, it is important that we build trust with the government, the schools, and with other partners in the community.

Reaction and Discussion[5]

Dr. Wong raised the issue of equity of care. He observed that *Crossing the Quality Chasm*, an Institute of Medicine report (IOM, 2001), mentioned equity as a critical aspect of ensuring quality health care in the United States. Traditionally, equity in health care has been related to performance measures, clinical outcomes, or the kind of the methodologies that are used with quality improvement. As a health care administrator, he asked, how do you view this domain of equity in how you are changing the models of what health care really is in your community?

When she thinks of equity in relation to her work at Southcentral, Ms. Gottlieb replied, she focuses on what it has done to target the Alaskan Native and American Indian populations. One-third of the funding South-

[5]The following discussions were edited and organized around major themes to provide a more readable summary and to eliminate duplication of topics.

central receives is from the Indian Health Service; another third comes from the state, foundations, and other grants; and the final third is earned as a result of existing aggressive building activities that were put in place after Southcentral took over management responsibilities from the federal government. Typically, as a government entity, any money generated by a third-party building would go back into the treasury. Yet as owners and managers, any funds that are generated from a third-party building can be distributed wherever money is needed to address health care disparities in the community. The Nation of Alaskan Natives and American Indians receives only one-third of the funding required for providing health care to the community from reimbursement from the federal government.

Dr. Levi raised the issue of sustainability. If community groups are asked to design programs that are sustainable, there is also an obligation on the part of the federal government and other funders to make sure that their funding streams are also sustainable. That is true for the Steps program and other programs as well. There have been discussions during the workshop about how communities need to integrate multiple funding streams into something that creates a true community-wide approach. However, he asked, do you think the current management of public health and health at the federal and state levels needs to change, so that the federal government creates a structure that makes it easier for people to reduce disparities at the local level?

Ms. Gottlieb replied that when the federal government began allocating funds to the Nation of Tribes under Public Law 9368, it did so in large lump sums. Money was allocated for emergency medical spending, primary care services, behavioral services, substance abuse, mental health, or other health care services. The allocation of funds determined how much money was put toward each of those health care needs. In 1997, however, the rules changed and the money began to be sent without a set allocation. Now when Southcentral receives a check for $45 million from the federal government, the tribal leadership can determine where those funds are most needed. This change has helped drive its success. Having power over the allocation of funds is the best way to address community needs.

Dr. Bracho shared her thoughts on partnerships. There are so many needs and so many jobs that need to be done to address the clinical concerns that partnering with other groups in other locations is incredibly challenging. It is extremely difficult to work on diabetes, obesity, or violence when they are associated with other issues, such as inadequate housing, lack of open space, or issues related to immigration reform. All of these issues need to be worked on simultaneously. Some of the examples discussed work more toward establishing partnerships to reach clinical goals rather than being hybrid models. If an organization partners with clinics and the government to improve diabetes management, but they do not tackle other issues related to poverty and inadequate housing, they are not necessarily hybrids, she noted.

Dr. Bracho also discussed issues related to community workers. Community workers live in the community and get paid to transform their communities, but they know that financing is needed for their community to improve. Now they are starting to be managed by members of academia and are receiving certification from people who know nothing about the communities that the workers represent. In this way, community workers are recognized as community leaders with implied credibility; yet, she asked, what type of community worker are they? How does one train and sustain them? In situations like this, the communities and the hybrid model are being forgotten.

Ms. Gottlieb responded that community health aides in Alaska are trained at the community level. The health aides are tribal people who receive training over a 6-month period, and they are often the only trained medical professionals in the entire village. That means that they are the doctor and the behaviorist. They provide all of the medical care in the community, and this system is working. It is simply impossible to provide a physician for $200,000 a year or more to every village.

Dr. Bracho countered that she would like to know what else is being done to rectify situations like the one in which Gottlieb's family used to live. What are you doing in your community to address issues like teen pregnancy or alcoholism? How are your health care strategies connected to the rest of the communities' efforts to follow a hybrid model, and how much are you doing to initiate change?

Ms. Gottlieb responded by discussing how funds are allocated in Alaska. Although there must be accountability, she said, she would still advocate for bulk funding, down to the level of those directly providing services. In receiving funds for providing a health care system, there must be accountability to the constituents who use those services. This means that funding would be allocated for community health workers if providing for these workers has been identified as a priority by the community.

REFERENCE

IOM (Institute of Medicine). 2001. Crossing the quality chasm: A new health system for the 21st century. Washington, DC: National Academy Press.

6

Moving Forward

The Roundtable on Health Disparities workshop set out to examine racial, ethnic, and geographic differentials in life expectancy in the United States; clinical and community-development approaches to reducing disparities; and implications of these approaches for developing actionable strategies. Throughout the workshop, Roundtable members and sponsors, presenters, and attendees discussed strategies, and shared opinions and suggestions, for making inroads into reducing health disparities. Their discussions focused on issues regarding data concerns, the importance of place, framing of the issue, racism, policy changes, fostering a broader spectrum of innovation, and funding. This chapter summarizes the salient points from the workshop presenters and participant's insights and reactions and provides initial steps for strategies to consider for moving forward.

DATA CONCERNS

Many workshop participants expressed their dissatisfaction with currently available data and worried about policy decisions being made that are based on existing inadequate or faulty data. Dr. Murray, the coauthor of "Eight Americas: Investigating Mortality Disparities Across Races, Counties, and Race-Counties in the United States" (see Appendix C), Dr. Acevedo-Garcia, of the Harvard School of Health, and Roundtable member Dr. Bracho suggested that more data should be collected and tracked at the county level so disparities and changing demographic patterns could be more accurately evaluated and monitored. Workshop participants also discussed the need for building information and data capacity in the United States.

Dr. Lawlor, coauthor of the paper "Community Approaches to Addressing Health Disparities" (see Appendix D), emphasized that in order for robust community-wide initiatives to be built and defended, there must be new community infrastructure and resources developed at the community level. He stressed that communities must bring together an array of social and economic data rather than relying on standard epidemiological data or health indicators alone. Very different traditional sources of data—racial, ethnic, and geographic data—will have to be brought together at the community level so that the health status of communities can be determined, and monitored and tracked, over time.

PLACE MATTERS

The presentations by Drs. Murray and Acevedo-Garcia stressed that where a person is raised or chooses to live will have a dramatic effect on their overall health and their access to quality health care. Dr. Murray presented his analyses using county-level mortality data, showing how life expectancies varied across the United States depending upon an individual's county of birth and emphasizing that people living in the United States have increased or decreased life expectancies depending on the geographic areas in which they live. Dr. Acevedo-Garcia also discussed the importance of place, but her presentation focused on U.S. metropolitan areas and how the impact of opportunity across neighborhoods affected the lives and health of the residents. Her presentation specifically emphasized the effect that neighborhood environments have on children and adolescents and how influences during these early stages of life can have long-term effects on their life course and, subsequently, on the long-term economic disparities extant in metropolitan areas.

FRAMING

Several workshop participants and members of the audience were concerned about finding a way to discuss or frame the issue of health disparities using methodologies and terminology that would resonate with policy makers and also capture the public's attention, both locally and nationally. Ms. Glover Blackwell, of PolicyLink, emphasized this point by suggesting that finding appropriate language for discussing these issues will ultimately determine whether or not there will ever be political and public will to be able to eliminate disparities. She also stressed that efforts to frame health disparities issues should not be limited to the realm of public or community health; they should include politicians, environmental health professionals, members of the general workforce, and people who work on housing issues.

Similar concerns were also expressed for framing issues pertaining to racism and institutional racism. Dr. Rhee, a Roundtable member, stressed that while the term health disparities may not resonate with the general public, terms such as *race* or *institutional racism* can be very powerful. He suggested that the language that is used to discuss these issues must be very forceful and specific, but it should not cause people to disengage or make them unwilling to join in the discussion to find solutions for these problems. Ms. Glover Blackwell agreed, adding that the appropriate words, strategies, and framing must be found that allow discussions to take place with key people at the table and in such a way that other people are invited into the discussion. There must be recognition that this is a charged discussion which cannot be approached in a way that isolates, accuses, or causes people to want to stay away.

Dr. Suggs, of the *St. Louis American*, suggested that discussions about racism should not focus solely on injustice but should also be considered in social and economic terms. He stressed that racial disparities are a disgrace, but they are also enormously expensive for this country. Ms. Schwartz, of the American College on Diversity, cautioned that all races and ethnicities are going to have to pay attention to the problems of racism and institutional racism because the demographics in the country are changing so rapidly and these issues will eventually affect everyone living in the United States.

CLINICAL AND COMMUNITY-BASED APPROACHES TO REDUCING DISPARITIES

During the workshop, Drs. Horowitz and Lawlor presented their paper "Community Approaches to Reducing Health Disparities," which assessed the implications for developing actionable strategies and describing methods of integrating clinical and community-based approaches to impacting communities and reducing health disparities. Hybrid models, which blend clinical and community-based approaches, should integrate community voices, community participation, and community ownership into disparities initiatives, emphasized Dr. Lawlor. They should also incorporate stakeholders from education, housing, employment, and other fundamental areas that are integral to the process of reducing disparities. Developing partnerships will be vital to the success of community initiatives, yet there needs to be a much broader understanding of who the relevant players should be and specifically who should be developing community-level initiatives.

Several workshop participants also stressed the importance of looking to international models for solutions to health disparities concerns in the

United States. Dr. Murray discussed how other developed countries around the globe have been able to succeed economically without experiencing the health disparities seen in the United States. He suggested that Americans are, in general, unwilling to want to learn from other countries' experiences. Several workshop participants agreed, including Dr. Levi, a member of the Roundtable, who stressed that the challenge is to find a way to frame health disparities issues in this country so that people recognize that a problem exists but to do so without making comparisons that could make people feel that the American way is inferior or that the proposed approach may not be a uniquely American approach. Dr. Lurie, the chair of the Roundtable, added that she would like to see models from less developed countries considered as well.

FUTURE INNOVATION

Workshop participants discussed several innovative ways to help reduce health disparities. Dr. Murray suggested that policies should be adopted that would foster a broader spectrum of innovation in addressing behavioral and pharmacologically manageable biological risks for noncommunicable diseases that also incorporates rigorous monitoring and ongoing evaluation. He believed that, with these measures in place, successful programs could be recognized, their results could be documented, and their methods could be shared and replicated.

Several workshop participants discussed policy changes that could take place within the United States to foster innovation. Dr. Murray and others discussed the importance of public–private partnerships being accompanied by significant resources, local applications, and the need for a strongly embedded monitoring and evaluation program to determine what is working as progress in this area is developing. He also suggested that many new strategies such as pay for performance, conditional cash transfers, or financial incentives are worth investigating. Dr. Lawlor discussed how existing community-development efforts, such as the Local Initiatives Support Corporation (LISC), or community-development investment banks could have a tremendous impact on the health of communities if they were to adopt health disparities concerns as a part of their agenda. Dr. Acevedo-Garcia suggested that modifying policies for Section 8 Voucher programs, fair housing enforcement, inclusionary zoning, and the availability of rental housing could help to reduce residential segregation and create more opportunities for low-income individuals and families.

Innovative international strategies should also be considered, suggested some workshop participants. The Global Alliance for Vaccines and Immunization (GAVI) was discussed by many workshop participants who praised the approach taken by GAVI for supporting innovative strategies for improving childhood immunization rates.

FUNDING

As was stated earlier, there are many domestic community development initiatives funding programs, such as LISC, that do not include health disparities concerns among the issues they address. Leveraging existing public–community partnerships and enacting policy changes that redirected their focus to include a health focus, suggested Dr. Lawlor, would have a dramatic impact on health disparities in the United States. Dr. Lawlor also suggested that potential sources of funding could include expanding support for Regional Health Commissions or creating collaborations between people who work on disparities issues and banks and corporations that support community-development initiatives so their collective knowledge and resources could have a greater impact on communities. He also suggested that university–community partnerships should be pursued, with the caveat that programs should be designed so that communities and the universities are both active participants in the planning process and that they work cooperatively to reach shared goals. Additionally, Dr. Lawlor suggested that the Roundtable could promote the idea of bringing together federal funding streams, such as those from the U.S. Department of Housing and Urban Development, so that money could be funneled to address specific areas of concern for disparities.

Ms. Glover Blackwell commented that there were many sources of funding for communities including after-school programs, youth development efforts, or community-development efforts such as LISC, but she suggested that communities should take ownership of that money and those programs because the funds being spent belong to the community and could be refocused to also reduce health disparities at the local level.

COMMUNITY INTERVENTION AND CAPACITY

Several presenters and members of the audience discussed the importance of community involvement in community-focused initiatives. Ms. Kubisch, a Roundtable member, stressed that power, money, resources, and political support are all necessary for driving community initiatives and suggested that community capacity is required at the organizational level in terms of being able to do the data analysis, community organizing, and advocacy to pull the funding streams together and have an impact on disparities.

Dr. Lawlor and Ms. Glover Blackwell suggested that organizations should exist in communities with the responsibility of gathering and interpreting community data so that there is a shared sense of what the challenges are, and that knowledge could be translated into compelling, relevant, and effective solutions. Ms. Glover Blackwell also suggested that there needs to be a public commitment to developing strategies to invest in new leadership and encourage young people to become leaders. She believes there should be a commitment to encourage potential leaders and provide them with opportunities to gain more exposure to mentors and to participate in commissions or other hands-on activities so they can become effective leaders in the future.

Several of the workshop presentations were presented by individuals who were coordinating local community initiatives or representing companies that are committed to reducing health disparities on a larger scale through education and advocacy. The representatives of Racial and Ethnic Approaches to Community Health (REACH) and Steps to a HealthierUS discussed their programs and shared successes and challenges that they have had while working to reduce disparities in their communities. Collectively, these presentations demonstrated that there are effective models to emulate and myriad examples of people who are directing programs that are producing results. The challenge going forward will be to implement programs like these on a national scale and learn how to successfully implement initiatives on a large scale.

CONCLUSION

The discussions at the workshop provided an opportunity for Roundtable members, presenters, and attendees to learn about several issues related to health disparities in the United States. The presentations and discourse on the importance of location of residence, framing, funding, data concerns, innovation, clinical and community-based approaches to reducing disparities, and community innovation and capacity, were helpful in providing several perspectives and viewpoints about what has been done, and what should take place in the future to reduce health disparities in the United States. The information gleaned from this workshop will help inform Roundtable members and workshop attendees so they can initiate, stimulate, or fund initiatives, take actions within their organizations, or share ideas and concepts from this workshop with other motivated stakeholders and partners. Through actions such as these, the workshop can be a catalyst for change and a means of moving closer to reaching the goal of eliminating health disparities.

Appendixes

Appendix A

Agenda of the Public Meeting Held by the Roundtable on Health Disparities

PUBLIC MEETING

Monday, July 30, 2007

The Bank of America Theater at Emerson Performance Center
Harris-Stowe State University
3026 Laclede Avenue
St. Louis, Missouri

8:45 am **WELCOME**
Dr. Henry Givens, President
Harris-Stowe State University

Nicole Lurie, Chair
Institute of Medicine Roundtable on Health Disparities

James R. Kimmey, President
Missouri Foundation for Health
Member, Institute of Medicine Roundtable on Health Disparities

9:00 am **Eight Americas: Investigating Mortality Disparities Across Races, Counties, and Race-Counties in the United States**
Christopher Murray, Professor of Global Health; Director, Institute for Health Metrics and Evaluation, University of Washington

9:45 am	**Panel Discussion: Implications of the Eight Americas Findings for Policy** *Dolores Acevedo-Garcia, Associate Professor* *Department of Society, Human Development and Health* *Harvard School of Public Health* *Donald Suggs, Publisher* *The St. Louis American* *Diane Schwartz* *President and CEO* *American Conference on Diversity* *William Dotson, Manager* *Health and Hospitals* *City of St. Louis*
10:30 am	**Audience Discussion**
11:30 am	**LUNCH—Board of Regents Gymnasium**
1:00 pm	**Clinical and Community-Development Approaches to Reducing Disparities** *Edward F. Lawlor, Dean* *George Warren Brown School of Social Work,* *Washington University in St. Louis* *Carol Horowitz, Assistant Professor* *Health Policy and Assistant Professor, Medicine* *Mt. Sinai University*
2:00 pm	**Successful Clinical and Community-Development Strategies** *Lisa Pivec, Director* *Community Health Promotion* *Cherokee Nation Health Services* *Janis E. Campbell, Principal Investigator* *Oklahoma REACH 2010* *Charmaine Ruddock, Project Director* *Bronx Health REACH*

3:00 pm **Panel Discussion: Implications of These Strategies for Developing Interventions**
Angela Glover Blackwell, Founder and Chief Executive Officer
PolicyLink

Nancy Williams, Acting Lead, Program Team
Steps to a HealthierUS Program Office
Centers for Disease Control and Prevention

Mary McFadden, Program Coordinator
Steps to a HealthierNY
Broome County Health Department

Katherine Gottlieb, President/CEO
Southcentral Foundation

4:00 pm **Audience Discussion: Ideas About Next Steps for the Roundtable**

4:30 pm **Wrap-Up**
Nicole Lurie, Chair
Institute of Medicine Roundtable on Health Disparities

5:00 pm **ADJOURN**

Appendix B

Workshop Presenters' Biosketches and Participant List

Dolores Acevedo-Garcia, Ph.D., MPA-URP, has a doctoral degree in public policy and demography (Princeton University, 1996). She is an associate professor in the Department of Society, Human Development and Health at the Harvard School of Public Health. Her research focuses on the effect of social determinants (e.g., residential segregation, immigrant adaptation) on health disparities along racial and ethnic lines; the role of nonhealth policies (e.g., housing policies, immigrant policies) in reducing those disparities; and the health and well-being of children with special needs and their families. Dr. Acevedo-Garcia is a member of the Social Science Advisory Board of the Poverty and Race Research Action Council. She is vice president of the Board of Directors of the Fair Housing Center of Greater Boston and chairs its Research Committee and she is a member of the Massachusetts Consortium for Children with Special Health Care Needs. Dr. Acevedo-Garcia is co-project director for DiversityData (http://diversitydata.sph.harvard.edu), an interactive website on socioeconomic indicators in U.S. metropolitan areas. DiversityData is an ongoing project of the Harvard School of Public Health and the Center for the Advancement of Health, supported by the W.K. Kellogg Foundation, and the Joint Center for Political and Economic Studies, Health Policy Institute. She is also co-founder and faculty mentor for the Interdisciplinary Consortium on Urban Planning and Public Health, an organization of students who have joined together around common interests at the intersection of the fields of public health and urban planning and design. With funding from the David Rockefeller Center for Latin American Studies at Harvard University, and the Kellogg Foundation, Dr. Acevedo-Garcia has led the creation of the Cross-national

Initiative on Place, Migration and Health, a diverse research network committed to understanding the links between migration processes and the health of (im)migrants, their families, and their sending and receiving communities using a cross-national lens for research and policy.

Angela Glover Blackwell, J.D., is founder and chief executive officer of PolicyLink, a national research and action institute that works collaboratively to develop and implement local, state, and federal policies to achieve economic and social equity. Previously, she was senior vice president at the Rockefeller Foundation. She also founded the Urban Strategies Council, a pioneering community-building organization in Oakland, California, and served as a partner with Public Advocates, a nationally known public interest law firm. She earned a bachelor's degree from Howard University and a law degree from the University of California, Berkeley.

Janis Campbell, Ph.D., is the surveillance coordinator for Chronic Disease at the Oklahoma State Department of Health. She has served in that position for 4 years. She has over 15 years experience with public health research and surveillance in Oklahoma. Dr. Campbell is the principal investigator for the Oklahoma Central Cancer Registry and the Oklahoma REACH 2010 Native American Project to Address Cardiovascular Disease and Diabetes. Dr. Campbell received her Ph.D. in anthropology in 1997 from the University of Oklahoma. Dr. Campbell is an adjunct faculty member at the Oklahoma University College of Public Health. She has published and presented locally and nationally on many occasions on topics related to health care among Native Americans in Oklahoma.

William (Bill) Dotson is chief of the Bureau of Family, School, and Community Health for the St. Louis Department of Health. He received his undergraduate degree from Webster University and graduate degrees in Clinical Psychology and Organizational Behavior from Washington University in St. Louis. He was also awarded an Honorary Ph.D. in Humanities from the University of Colorado for his HIV/AIDS work in minority communities. Mr. Dotson is a founding appointee to the Minority Health Advisory Committee in the State of Missouri Department of Health, and a founding Mayoral appointee and co-chair to the Ryan White Planning Council for the City of St. Louis. With over 15 years of public health service as a manager and educator for the City of St. Louis Department of Health, Mr. Dotson has had responsibility for developing community collaborations, securing funding, and implementing initiatives designed to impact critical health disparities in the City of St. Louis. He is also a distinguished lecturer on minority health.

Katherine Gottlieb has an M.B.A. from Alaska Pacific University and has been President/CEO of the Southcentral Foundation since 1987. Under her leadership, Southcentral Foundation has grown from fewer than 100 employees to more than 1,200 and from an annual operating budget of about $3 million to one of $100 million. It provides more than 65 medical and behavioral health services programs. Ms. Gottlieb is of Aleut descent, and is a member of CIRI, which is 1 of 12 in-state Native regional corporations established by Congress under the terms of the Alaska Native Claims Settlement Act.

Carol Horowitz, M.D., M.P.H., is an assistant professor in the Departments of Health Policy and Medicine at the Mount Sinai School of Medicine in New York City. As a primary care physician and health services researcher, her primary interest is in understanding and eliminating racial and ethnic disparities using community-based participatory research methods. Currently, she directs the East Harlem Diabetes Center of Excellence, a community-based coalition with a goal to better the lives of individuals with diabetes. She is also the principal investigator of a National Institutes of Health (NIH) grant, and of the Community Core of an NIH-funded center, both of which aim to improve chronic disease outcomes amongst residents of Harlem, New York City, through community-based research interventions. She received her B.S. and M.D. from Cornell University, trained in internal medicine and primary care at the Albert Einstein School of Medicine in the Bronx, and was a Robert Wood Johnson Clinical Scholar at the University of Washington in Seattle.

Edward F. Lawlor, Ph.D., holds a B.A. in economics, government, and legal studies from Bowdoin College. He received his Ph.D. from the Florence Heller Graduate School for Advanced Studies in Social Welfare at Brandeis University. He is currently the dean and William E. Gordon Professor at the George Warren Brown School of Social Work at Washington University in St. Louis. Professor Lawlor has published widely on access to health care, health care reform, policy analysis, and aging. He is the author of *Redesigning the Medicare Contract: Politics, Markets, and Agency* and founding editor of the *Public Policy and Aging Report.*

Mary McFadden received a B.A. in health science from State University of New York at Cortland in 1988, began a career in public health at the Broome County Public Health Department with the Women, Infants, and Children's program as a public health representative in 1991, and was instrumental for developing and implementing the first WIC Breastfeeding Peer Counseling program in Broome County. In addition, she was instrumental in the development and incorporation of the Southern Tier Breastfeeding Coalition. In 1996 she was promoted to a public health educator for the Cancer Services program, and in 1998 promoted to supervising public health educator to implement and oversee an integrated chronic disease risk reduction program. In 2000, Ms. McFadden received the New York State Department of Health's Partner of Distinction Award. In September 2003 to the present, she has overseen the Steps to a HealthierNY program in Broome County. Ms. McFadden has presented the successes of Broome County's Steps program around the Country, including the U.S. Department of Health and Human Services' Office of Disease Prevention and Health Promotion and the Centers for Disease Control Annual National Prevention Summit. Lastly, and most importantly, she is the mother of two young boys who provide her with the ultimate challenge of her health education expertise.

Christopher J. L. Murray, D.Phil., M.D., is the director of the Institute for Health Metrics and Evaluation at the University of Washington and Professor of Global Health at the University of Washington School of Medicine. A physician and health economist, his early work focused on tuberculosis control and the development with Dr. Alan Lopez of the Global Burden of Disease methods and applications. In this work, they developed a new metric to compare death and disability from various diseases and the contribution of risk factors to the overall burden of disease in developing and developed countries. This pioneering effort has been hailed as a major landmark in public health and an important foundation for policy formulation and priority setting. He has also contributed to the development of a range of new methods and empirical studies to strengthen the basis for population health measurement and cost-effectiveness analysis. He worked at the World Health Organization from 1998 to 2003 where he served as the Executive Director of the Evidence and Information for Policy Cluster while Gro Harlem Brundtland was Director-General. Since 1998, a main thrust of his work has been on the conceptualization, measurement, and application of approaches to understand the inputs, organization, outputs, and outcomes of health systems. From 2003 until 2007, he was the director of the Harvard University Initiative for Global Health and the Richard Saltonstall Professor of Public Policy. Dr. Murray has authored or edited 14 books, many book chapters, and more than 120 journal articles in internationally peer-reviewed publications. He holds a B.A. from Harvard College, a D.Phil. from Oxford University, and an M.D. from Harvard Medical School.

Lisa Pivec is the Director of Community Health Promotion for Cherokee Nation Health Services. She holds a master's degree from Northeastern State University in college teaching with an emphasis in health. Ms. Pivec has been with the Cherokee Nation since 1991 and currently works closely with the Oklahoma State Department of Health REACH 2010 project, the Centers for Disease Control and Prevention Steps to a HealthierUS and Tobacco Control Tribal Support Center projects, and she chairs the Cherokee Nation Community Health Services Committee. Ms. Pivec is a member of the Cherokee Nation and is originally from the Peavine community in Adair County. She hopes to continue working with and for Cherokee people throughout her career.

Charmaine Ruddock, M.S., project director, Bronx Health REACH, the Institute for Urban Family Health, has been involved in the administration of health care services to medically underserved communities for more than 10 years, notably in the design, development, and operational oversight of Medicaid Managed Care Organizations serving communities in New York City, Long Island, and Connecticut. She has sat on the Board of Directors of the New York Prenatal Care Steering Committee and HHFII, organizations dedicated to improving the health outcomes of New Yorkers. Ms. Ruddock joined the Institute for Urban Family Health in 2000 to direct Bronx Health REACH, a coalition of 40 community- and faith-based organizations, funded by the Centers for Disease Control REACH 2010 initiative. In addition to REACH, Ms. Ruddock also directs two other diabetes-focused initiatives—the Diabetes Prevention and Control Initiative funded by the New York State Department of Health Bureau of Chronic Diseases Services and an NIH-funded initiative exploring the use of faith-based organizations to provide diabetes education. Bronx Health REACH's goal is the elimination of racial and ethnic disparities in health outcomes in the southwest Bronx. The health priority focus is diabetes and heart disease. Ms. Ruddock is working with several community groups, faith-based organizations, and health care providers to implement several initiatives, namely the Primary Prevention and Public Health Education Program; Community Health Advocacy; Faith-Based Outreach efforts; a Legal and Regulatory workgroup; and the Grocer and Restaurant Outreach Program. Ms. Ruddock holds a bachelor's degree in literature and social sciences from the University of the West Indies and a masters of science in management and policy analysis from the Graduate School of Management, The New School for Social Research.

Diane Schwartz is the president and CEO of the American Conference on Diversity. Ms. Schwartz manages the American Conference on Diversity's community, program, public relations, and marketing functions throughout the State of New Jersey. She has over 25 years of experience in the field. Ms. Schwartz holds a B.A. and M.A. in English from Monmouth University and has done postgraduate work in marketing. A published author, her articles on health care, management, and human relations issues have appeared in national and state publications. With over 25 years of experience in creating and implementing organizational development programs for nonprofit groups in the state, she has revitalized and expanded community groups and organizations to maximize their potential. For years, Ms. Schwartz produced and hosted Healthview, a half-hour television information program airing weekly on CTN of New Jersey. She has appeared on numerous television programs sharing information and expertise on human relations issues. She is an active participant in the community as a member of the NJN-New Jersey Public Television Diversity in Action Committee and as a member of the New Jersey Human Relations Council Advisory Board. Ms. Schwartz is also a member of the Monmouth County Human Relations Commission and has served on the Long Range Planning Committee for the New Jersey Commission on Higher Education. She is a member of the Board of Directors of Leadership New Jersey and was a Fellow of Leadership New Jersey, Class of 2002. She is a member of the Executive Women of New Jersey. Prior to joining the American Conference on Diversity, Ms. Schwartz was Senior Vice President of Public Affairs for Raritan Bay Health Services Corporation, a two-hospital, multifaceted health care system in central New Jersey, and she also managed the Raritan Bay Healthcare Foundation. She has served variously as president of both the Perth Amboy and Old Bridge Chambers of Commerce; president of the Perth Amboy Rotary, where she was honored as a Paul Harris Fellow; and as a director of the Woodbridge Metro Chamber of Commerce. She is a past chair of the Business Coalition for Perth Amboy Youth, a coalition of business, education, and municipal representatives developing jobs for urban youth. She served as a director of Camp Kiddie Keep Well, a New Jersey camp for underprivileged children. She was a member of the Mayor's Economic Development Committee for the City of Perth Amboy, and was on the Marketing Committee of the Old Bridge Economic Development Corporation. In 1992, the Perth Amboy Chamber of Commerce named her Executive of the Year. Ms. Schwartz is former vice president of the Hospital Fund Raising Executives of New Jersey, a past president of the New Jersey Hospital Public Relations and Marketing Association, and a featured speaker and consultant for various business, industry, and nonprofit organizations throughout the region. Ms. Schwartz is married and has four grown children. She and her husband live in Colts Neck, New Jersey.

Donald M. Suggs, D.D.S., was born in East Chicago, Indiana, and attended the public schools there. He graduated with B.S. and D.D.S. degrees from Indiana University, then did his postgraduate work at Washington University Dental School and Homer G. Phillips Hospital. He served as chief of oral surgery at Dover Air Force Base in Delaware and was the first African

American to serve as an associate clinical professor at St. Louis University Dental School. Dr. Suggs was a fellow of the American Association of Oral and Maxillo-Facial Surgeons and has a limited private practice in his specialty. Active in the Civil Rights Movement in the 1960s and 1970s, he served as chairman of the Poor People's March-on-Washington in 1968. Later, he became founder and chairman of the African Continuum, organized to bring serious noncommercial African American artistic endeavors to St. Louis. He was a long-time president of the Alexander-Suggs Gallery of African Art based in St. Louis and New York City (1970–1989). He is a founding member of the Center for African Art (now the Museum of African Art in New York City) and is a former member of the board of directors of the Studio Museum in New York. Dr. Suggs currently serves on the St. Louis Art Museum Board of Commissioners. He was the first African American to serve as president of the Convention and Visitors Bureau of St. Louis. His business activities also include president of Arch Concessions and a partner with D & D Concessions and the City Plaza Project. Dr. Suggs has been awarded honorary doctorate degrees from the University of Missouri-St. Louis, Harris-Stowe State University, and St. Louis University and is the recipient of many civic awards. He is currently president and publisher of the *St. Louis American Newspaper*, Missouri's largest black newspaper. He is the father of Donald M. Jr., Dawn Marie, and Dina Margaret.

Captain Nancy Williams has been working in public health for over 30 years. She has been with the U.S. Public Health Service for 23 years, working in the Indian Health Service and the Centers for Disease Control and Prevention (CDC). She received her MSPH from the University of Massachusetts at Amherst. She has worked as the first Tribal Health Educator for the Hopi Tribe, with the Arizona Department of Health, and the San Bernardino County Health Department. While in the Indian Health Service, she worked in the Albuquerque, Phoenix, and Nashville areas. She spent 2 years detailed to the Department of the Interior working with the Commonwealth of the Northern Marianas Islands. While at CDC, she worked with the Office on Smoking and Health, and the Steps to a HealthierUS Program Office, where she is presently the acting lead for the Program Team.

PARTICIPANT LIST

Dara Autumn
Missouri Foundation for Health
St. Louis, MO

RADM John Babb
Department of Health and Human Services
Kansas City, MO

Ryan Barker
Missouri Foundation for Health
St. Louis, MO

Caroline Battles
Missouri Foundation for Health
St. Louis, MO

CAPT Jose Belardo
Department of Health and Human Services
Kansas City, MO

Judy Bentley
Community Health-In-Partnership Services (CHIPS)
St. Louis, MO

Rudy Bess
Hope Light Foundation
Hazelwood, MO

Sarah Betsworth
St. Louis University
School of Public Health
St. Louis, MO

Angela Bowman, MSW, PLCSW
Bi-Lingual International Assistant Services
St. Louis, MO

Gloria Brand
OWH Department of Health and Human Services
Jefferson City, MO

Marilyn Brown
St. Louis University
School of Public Health
St. Louis, MO

Moira Cahan
Missouri Foundation for Health
St. Louis, MO

Aurita Caldwell
Department of Health and Human Services
St. Louis, MO

James Campbell
Oklahoma State Department of Health
Oklahoma City, OK

Maria E. Cepeda, MHA
Office of Minority Health Department of Health and Senior Services
Jefferson City, MO

Catrina Chambers, MSPH
St. Louis University
St. Louis, MO

Siobhan Champ-Blackwell, MSLIS
National Network of Libraries of Medicine, Midcontinental Region
Creighton University Health
Omaha, NE

Debbie Chase
Clayton, MO

Leann Chilton
Barnes-Jewish Healthcare
St. Louis, MO

Arthur Colbert
Missouri Foundation for Health
St. Louis, MO

LaVonda Cotton
Williams & Associates, Inc.
St. Louis, MO

Ana-Paula Cupertino, PhD
University of Kansas Medical Center
Kansas City, KS

L. Dauernheim
St. Louis, MO

Jesse DeLeon
Southeast Missouri Health Network
Kennett, MO

Mary Deverman
Cenlene Foundation for Quality Healthcare
Clayton, MO

Margaret Donnelly
State Representative
St. Louis, MO

Monica Dykas
Interfaith Partnership
St. Louis, MO

Kate Eddens
St. Louis University
School of Public Health
St. Louis, MO

Bert Emmons
Sober Living-Midwest
St. Louis, MO

Jannis Evans
Office of Minority Health
Jefferson City, MO

Angela Fleming, MPH
Interfaith Partnership of Metropolitan
St. Louis/Faith Beyond Walls
St. Louis, MO

Ben Francisco, PhD, PNP, AE-C
University of Missouri, Columbia

Vannessa Frazier
Howardville Community Betterment
Howardville, MO

Alicia Galan
Department of Health and Human Services, Office for Civil Rights, Region VII
Kansas City, MO

CAPT Edwin Galan
Department of Health and Human Services
Kansas City, MO

Toni Garrison, MHA
Passport Health—The Vaccine People
St. Louis, MO

Elizabeth George
Deacon Foundation
St. Louis, MO

Hannah Gilk
Institute of Family Medicine
St. Louis, MO

James E. Green
Williams & Associates, Inc.
St. Louis, MO

Deidre Griffith
St. Louis University
School of Public Health
St. Louis, MO

Rosalind Guy
St. Louis, MO

Sandi Leland Hawk
St. Louis Maternal, Child and
Family Health Coalition
St. Louis, MO

Cynthia Hayes
Missouri Foundation for Health
St. Louis, MO

Kym Hemley
SOCF
Cleveland, OH

Rich Hennicke
Nurses for Newborns Foundation
St. Louis, MO

Warren Holloman, Jr.
Williams & Associates, Inc.
St. Louis, MO

Mary E. Homan, MA
St. Louis University
School of Public Health
St. Louis, MO

Ellen Horan
Catholic Health Association
St. Louis, MO

William Hudson
Freelance Writer
St. Louis, MO

Betty Kao
St. Louis Christian Chinese
Community Service Center
St Louis, MO

Rosetta Keeton
St. Louis ConnectCare Community
Health Centers
St. Louis, MO

Pamela Kelly, MBA
Missouri Telehealth Network
St. Louis, MO

Yit Mui Khoo
St. Louis Christian Chinese
Community Service Center
St Louis, MO

Karley M. King
Chesterfield, MO

Hope Krebill
National Cancer Institute's Cancer
Information Service
Kansas City, KS

Christy Lapka
St. Louis University
School of Public Health
St. Louis, MO

Johnnie Miller Matlock
St. Louis, MO

Joe McCarthy
Missouri Foundation for Health
St. Louis, MO

Martin McCrary
St. Louis, MO

Joan McGivney
St. Louis, MO

Joris Miller
Community Alternatives
St. Louis, MO

Margie Minor
OMH—Department of Health and Human Services
St. Louis, MO

Carolyn Montgomery
Southeast Missouri Health Network
Portageville, MO

Bobbi Morris
Southeast Missouri University
Cape Girardeau, MO

Ibrahim A. Muhammad
Muhammad Blamic Academy
St. Louis, MO

Saffiyah Muhammad
Hazelwood, MO

E. Rachel Mutrux
Missouri Telehealth Network
Unversity of Missouri School of Medicine
Columbia, MO

Marcia Newton
St. Louis City Health Department
St. Louis, MO

Warren Nichols
St. Louis Department of Health
St. Louis, MO

Akihiko Noudin
St. Louis University
St. Louis, MO

Sandy Ortia
Southeast Missouri University
Cape Girardeau, MO

Bev Pfeifer-Harms
Missouri Foundation for Health
St. Louis, MO

David Pfieffer
St. Louis University
School of Public Health
St. Louis, MO

Debbie Pfeiffer, MA
St. Louis University
School of Public Health
St. Louis, MO

Nancy Phillips, MSW, LCSW
Midtown Catholic Charities Community Services
St. Louis, MO

Salim Phillips
Williams & Associates, Inc.
St. Louis, MO

Terry Plain
Missouri Foundation for Health
St. Louis, MO

Cynthia L. Price
Southern Illinois Healthcare Foundation
St. Louis, MO

Evelyn Pullian
Southeast Missouri Health Network
Kennett, MO

Gwen Ratermann
Center for Health Policy
University of Missouri
Columbia, MO

Leslie Reed
Missouri Foundation for Health
St. Louis, MO

Evelyn Reid
Webster University
St. Louis, MO

Karen Roth
St. Louis Business Health Coalition
St. Louis, MO

Mitch Schneider
West End Word
St Louis, MO

Lisa Schwarb
University of Missouri
Columbia, MO

Deena Scott
Missouri Foundation for Health
St. Louis, MO

Donna Shoff
Missouri Foundation for Health
St. Louis, MO

Linda Spinn
Nurses for Newborns Foundation
St. Louis, MO

Jill Thompson
Maternal Child & Family Health Coalition
St. Louis, MO

Vetta L. Thompson
St. Louis University
St. Louis, MO

Donna Vent
Southeast Missouri Health Network
New Madrid, MO

Eduardo J. Vera
Language Access Metro Project (LAMP) an Agency of Catholic Family Services
St. Louis, MO

Heather Weeden
St. Louis, MO

Consuelo Hopkins Wilkins, MD
Washington University School of Medicine
St. Louis, MO

Erise Williams
Williams & Associates, Inc.
St. Louis, MO

Paula E. Wills
Health Visions of East St. Louis
East St. Louis, IL

Jennifer Wood
Missouri Foundation for Health
St. Louis, MO

Appendix C

Eight Americas: Investigating Mortality Disparities Across Races, Counties, and Race-Counties in the United States[1]

Christopher J. L. Murray,[2] Sandeep C. Kulkarni,[3] Catherine Michaud,[4] Niels Tomijima,[5] Maria T. Bulzacchelli,[6] Terrell J. Iandiorio,[7] Majid Ezzat

Funding: This research was supported by a cooperative agreement, awarded by the Centers for Disease Control and Prevention and the Association of Schools of Public Health (grant U36/CCU300430–23) and by the National Institute on Aging (grant PO1AG17625). The funders had no role in study design, data collection and analysis, decision to publish, or preparation of the manuscript. The contents of this article are solely the responsibility of the authors and do not necessarily represent the official views of the Centers for Disease Control and Prevention or the Association of Schools of Public Health.

---

[1]Reprinted, with permission, from *PLoS Medicine*, http://medicine.plosjournals.org/perlserv/?SESSID=d0a2681557eece4143f1a664d5536f5f&request=get-document&doi=10.1371/journal.pmed.0030260.

[2]Harvard School of Public Health, Harvard University Initiative for Global Health, and Center for Population and Development Studies, Harvard University, Cambridge, Massachusetts.

[3]Harvard University Initiative for Global Health, Cambridge, Massachusetts, and University of California San Francisco, San Francisco, California.

[4]Harvard University Initiative for Global Health, and Center for Population and Development Studies, Harvard University, Cambridge, Massachusetts.

[5]Center for Population and Development Studies, Harvard University, Cambridge, Massachusetts.

[6]Center for Population and Development Studies, Harvard University, Cambridge, Massachusetts.

[7]Center for Population and Development Studies, Harvard University, Cambridge, Massachusetts.

Competing Interests: The authors have declared that no competing interests exist.

Academic Editor: Thomas Novotny, University of California San Francisco.

Citation: Murray CJL, Kulkarni SC, Michaud C, Tomijima N, Bulzacchelli MT, et al. (2006) Eight Americas: Investigating mortality disparities across races, counties, and race-counties in the United States. PLoS Med 3(9): e260. DOI: 10.1371/journal.pmed.0030260.

Received: October 17, 2005
Accepted: March 31, 2006
Published: September 12, 2006

DOI: 10.1371/journal.pmed.0030260

Abbreviations: BRFSS, Behavioral Risk Factor Surveillance System; NCHS, National Center for Health Statistics; SES, socioeconomic status.

ABSTRACT

Background

The gap between the highest and lowest life expectancies for race-county combinations in the United States is over 35 y. We divided the race-county combinations of the US population into eight distinct groups, referred to as the "eight Americas," to explore the causes of the disparities that can inform specific public health intervention policies and programs.

Methods and Findings

The eight Americas were defined based on race, location of the county of residence, population density, race-specific county-level per capita income, and cumulative homicide rate. Data sources for population and mortality figures were the Bureau of the Census and the National Center for Health Statistics. We estimated life expectancy, the risk of mortality from specific diseases, health insurance, and health-care utilization for the eight Americas. The life expectancy gap between the 3.4 million high-risk urban black males and the 5.6 million Asian females was 20.7 y in 2001. Within the sexes, the life expectancy gap between the best-off and the worst-off groups was 15.4 y for males (Asians versus high-risk urban blacks) and 12.8 y for females (Asians versus low-income southern rural blacks). Mortality disparities among the eight Americas were largest for young (15–44 y) and middle-aged (45–59 y) adults, especially for men. The disparities were caused primarily by a number of chronic diseases and injuries with well-established risk factors. Between 1982 and 2001, the ordering of life expectancy among the eight Americas and the absolute difference between the advantaged and disadvantaged groups remained largely unchanged. Self-reported health plan coverage was lowest for western Native Americans and low-income southern rural blacks. Crude self-reported health-care utilization, however, was slightly higher for the more disadvantaged populations.

Conclusions

Disparities in mortality across the eight Americas, each consisting of millions or tens of millions of Americans, are enormous by all international standards. The observed disparities in life expectancy cannot be explained by race, income, or basic health-care access and utilization alone. Because policies aimed at reducing fundamental socioeconomic inequalities are currently practically absent in the US, health disparities will have to be at least partly addressed through public health strategies that reduce risk factors for chronic diseases and injuries.

The Editors' Summary of this article follows the references.

INTRODUCTION

Health disparities in the United States have been the subject of extensive critical scrutiny and analysis. Multiple investigations have documented the consistent gap in all measures of mortality by race, particularly between black and white Americans [1–5]. Researchers have also drawn attention to substantial disparities in mortality and functional health status nationally and within race groups in relation to income, social class, education, and community characteristics [6–16]. Inequalities in insurance coverage, health-care access and utilization, and more recently in quality of care have also been investigated [17–22]. The Department of Health and Human Services has launched its Initiative to Eliminate Racial and Ethnic Disparities in Health, with programs focused on a number of diseases including cardiovascular disease, HIV, and diabetes.

Life expectancy by race in the US in 2001 ranged from 86.7 for Asian females to 68.7 for black males, a gap of 18 y. Analysis of life expectancy by county of residence and by the combination of race and county of residence (referred to as "race-county" in this paper) demonstrates even larger disparities [23]. County-level analysis of mortality for 1997–2001 (pooled over 5 y to increase sample size) demonstrates a 22.5-y gap in life expectancy between males in southwest South Dakota and females in Stearns County, Minnesota (see Dataset S1 for life expectancy by county). When race-county combinations are considered, life expectancy disparities are dramatically larger. For example, Native American males in the cluster of Bennet, Jackson, Mellette, Shannon, Todd, and Washabaugh Counties in South Dakota had a life expectancy of 58 y in 1997–2001, compared to Asian females in Bergen County, New Jersey, with a life expectancy of 91 y, a gap of 33 y (see also Figure 1). Mortality inequalities in subgroups within race-counties, such as those defined based on socioeconomic status (SES), may be even larger. Because of small sample size and the absence of individual-level linked data needed to study race-county-SES combinations, it is currently not possible to study mortality patterns within race groups in small geographic areas, or even states. The largest measurable gaps observed in the US to-date are those revealed by examining the inequalities across race-county groups.

Formulating effective policies and programs to ameliorate health inequalities requires an understanding of the interrelated causes of mortality disparities, specific interventions to mitigate these causes, and intervention delivery mechanisms [24,25]. Efforts to characterize the contributions of specific diseases and injuries, risk factors such as tobacco, alcohol, or obesity, access to effective health care, and the broader socioeconomic determinants of health and disease are severely hampered by data limitations: the analysis of mortality by age and disease for specific race-counties is affected by the small numbers of deaths, such that even pooling data for 10 y or more does not provide sufficient person-years of observation to draw stable and robust conclusions for some diseases, especially by age. Data on risk factor exposure and health-care access and utilization are even more limited, as there are almost no sources of information on these variables by race and county.

In order to investigate the causes of the observed race-county mortality disparities, within the limitations posed by sample size, we have divided US race-counties into eight subgroups based on a number of sociodemographic and geographical variables, referred to as the "eight Americas." In addition to examining the role of specific diseases in age-specific and all-age mortality disparities, the eight Americas analysis identifies distinct subgroups, based on a small number of sociodemographic and geographical indicators, towards whom public health and medical interventions may be targeted. We emphasize that the grouping of US race-counties into the eight Americas in our analysis is not the only division that could be used for understanding the large mortality inequalities across racecounties. This grouping however reveals important variations in total as well as age-, sex-, and disease-specific mortality that call for further investigation of causes and potential interventions.

METHODS

Definition of the Eight Americas

We estimated life expectancy for eight subgroups of the US population, which we refer to as the "eight Americas." The building blocks for the eight Americas were a combination of race and county of residence. The race-county units were combined based on a number of socioeconomic and geographical indicators, including the location of the county of residence, population density, race-specific county-level per capita income, and cumulative homicide rate (Table 1; Figure 2).

We arranged the 3,141 US counties into 2,072 individual or merged county units. There were two reasons for forming merged county units. (1) To avoid very small county populations and numbers of deaths, smaller counties were merged with adjacent counties to form units with total population of at least 10,000 males and 10,000 females. (2) Merged county units were also formed where necessary to account for changes in county status and county lines, such as formations of new counties and incorporation of independent cities (which are officially equivalent to counties) into surrounding counties. The result was a consistent set of 2,072 individual or merged county units that represent the same physical land areas from 1980 through the present. We then divided the entire US population (the race-county units) into eight distinct subgroups, the eight Americas, based on the location of the county of residence, population density, per capita income of the county of residence in 1990, and cumulative homicide rate (averaged between 1991 and 2001 to reduce sensitivity to outlier years) (Table 1; Figure 2). We used a population density of greater than 100 persons/km^2 to distinguish urban from rural areas. Low-income race-county combinations were defined as those below the national median of race-specific county-level per capita income. Cumulative homicide rate was used as an indicator of deterioration of social institutions and neighborhood cohesion. These factors have been found to adversely affect health outcomes above and beyond individual characteristics [26,27]. High-risk urban areas were defined as those where the cumulative probability of homicide death between the ages of 15 and 74 exceeded the 95th percentile of all US counties, or 1.1%.

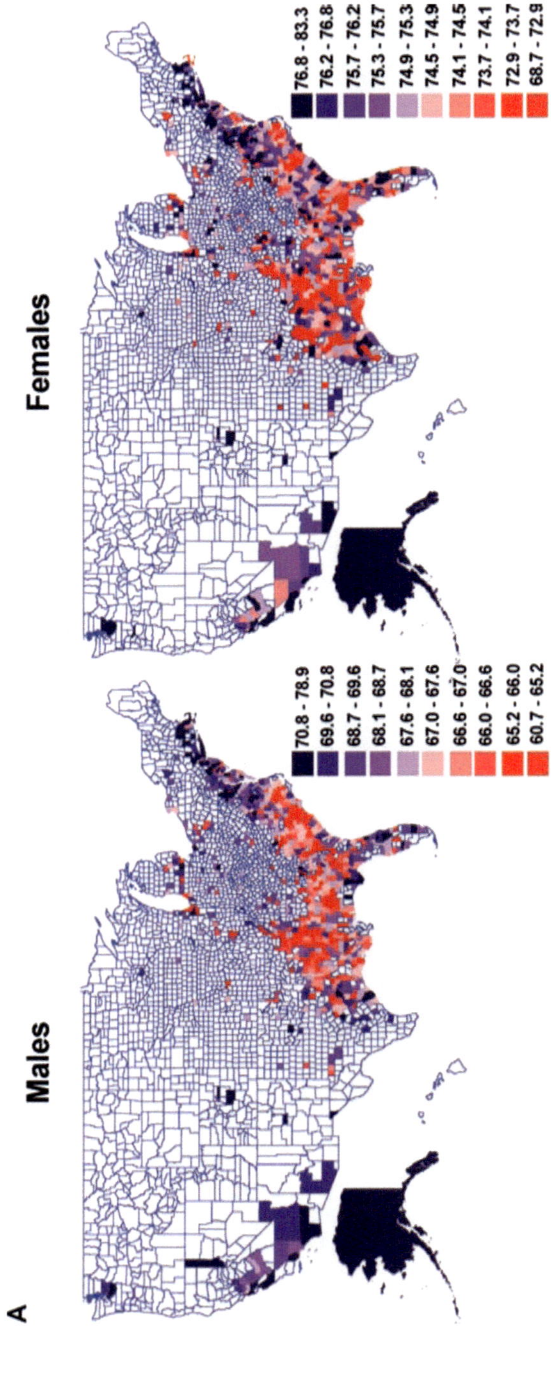
A
Males
70.8 - 78.9
69.6 - 70.8
68.7 - 69.6
68.1 - 68.7
67.6 - 68.1
67.0 - 67.6
66.6 - 67.0
66.0 - 66.6
65.2 - 66.0
60.7 - 65.2
Females
76.8 - 83.3
76.2 - 76.8
75.7 - 76.2
75.3 - 75.7
74.9 - 75.3
74.5 - 74.9
74.1 - 74.5
73.7 - 74.1
72.9 - 73.7
68.7 - 72.9

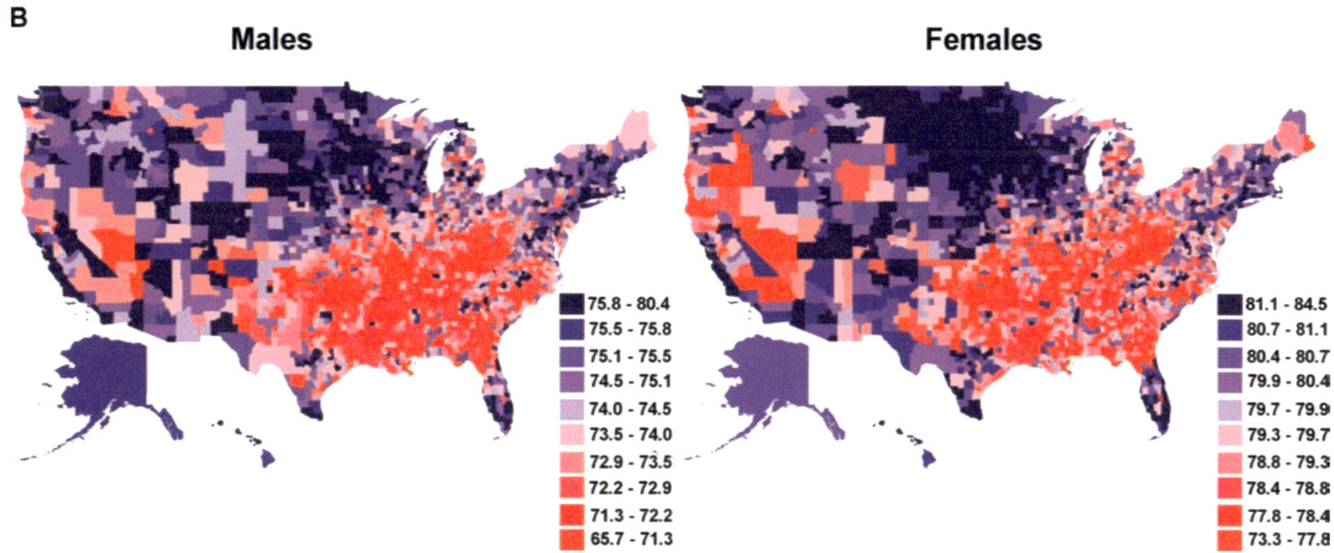

Figure 1. County Life Expectancies by Race

Deaths were averaged for 1997–2001 to reduce sensitivity to small numbers and outliers.

(A) Life expectancy at birth for black males and females. Only counties with more than five deaths for any 5-y age group (0–85) were mapped, to avoid unstable results.

(B) Life expectancy at birth for white males and females.

DOI: 10.1371/journal.pmed.0030260.g001

Table 1. Definitions and Basic Sociodemographic Characteristics of the Eight Americas

America	General Description	Population (Millions)	Average Income Per Capita	Percent Completing High School	Definition
1	Asian	10.4	$21,566	80%	Asians living in counties where Pacific Islanders make up less than 40% of total Asian population
2	Northland low-income rural white	3.6	$17,758	83%	Whites in northern plains and Dakotas with 1990 county-level per capita income below $11,775 and population density less than 100 persons/km^2
3	Middle America	214.0	$24,640	84%	All other whites not included in Americas 2 and 4, Asians not in America 1, and Native Americans not in America 5
4	Low-income whites in Appalachia and the Mississippi Valley	16.6	$16,390	72%	Whites in Appalachia and the Mississippi Valley with 1990 county-level per capita income below $11,775
5	Western Native American	1.0	$10,029	69%	Native American populations in the mountain and plains areas, predominantly on reservations
6	Black Middle America	23.4	$15,412	75%	All other black populations living in countries not included in Americas 7 and 8
7	Southern low-income rural black	5.8	$10,463	61%	Blacks living in counties in the Mississippi Valley and the Deep South with population density below 100 persons/km^2, 1990 county-level per capita income below $7,500, and total population size above 1,000 persons (to avoid small numbers)
8	High-risk urban black	7.5	$14,800	72%	Urban populations of more than 150,000 blacks living in counties with cumulative probability of homicide death between 15 and 74 y greater than 1.0%

Population, income per capita, and education were calculated for race-county combinations from the 2000 US census.
DOI: 10.1371/journal.pmed.0030260.t001

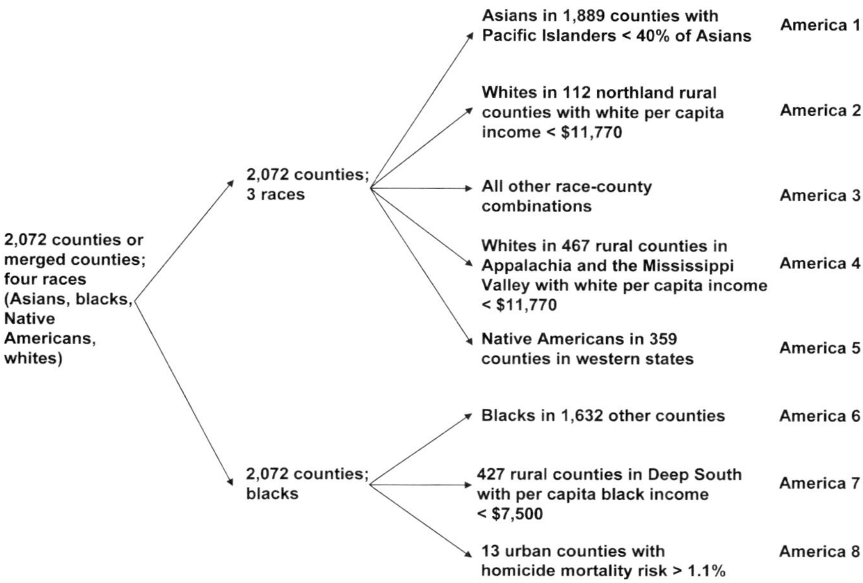

Figure 2. Construction of the Eight Americas from 8,288 Race-County Units
DOI: 10.1371/journal.pmed.0030260.g002

Data Sources for Population, Mortality, and Sociodemographic Indicators

Bureau of the Census population estimates and National Center for Health Statistics bridged-race population estimates.

For 1982–1989, we interpolated age-, sex-, race-, and county-specific population figures using the 1980 and 1990 censual figures, assuming a constant growth rate. For 1990–2001, we used the bridged-race population estimates, released by the National Center for Health Statistics (NCHS), to be consistent with race categories used in mortality registration [28]. Race was defined according to the 1977 US Office of Management and Budget definition of the four race groups (Asians, blacks, Native Americans, and whites), which has been preserved in the bridged and censual population estimates. Race-specific county income was from the 1990 census [29].

NCHS mortality statistics.

All deaths occurring in the US are reported to the NCHS, with causes of deaths coded to follow the International Classification of Disease system. NCHS data also include county of residence (matched to the US census), race, sex, and age. Public-use mortality files, available through the

NCHS [30] or the National Bureau of Economic Research, do not provide county identifiers for deaths in counties with fewer than 100,000 people. We obtained county identifiers for all deaths for years 1982 through 2001 through a special request to the NCHS. County identifiers for years after 2002 were not provided to us because of changes in NCHS policy. NCHS race categories were collapsed into the four Office of Management and Budget categories. A very small proportion (<0.001%) of all deaths were classified as "other race." We assumed these deaths to be among Asians, the group with the best mortality experience, in order not to overestimate disparities.

Despite the fact that we used the NCHS bridged-race population estimates, which are estimated for consistency of race definitions with those in death certificates and mortality statistics, there may be differential under- or overestimation of race-specific population and mortality. This can occur because race is recorded by individuals or their families in the census (population) and by the certifying physician or funeral facility on the death certificate (mortality). This differential recording system is a potential source of bias in life expectancy, especially for the smaller race groups: Native Americans and Asians [1,31]. The bias for Native Americans observed in national data is unlikely to affect our estimates because the grouping used in the eight Americas distinguishes those Native Americans who primarily live on or near reservations (America 5), and are hence less likely to be undercounted, from the remaining Native Americans, who are included in America 3. For Asians, this source of bias was addressed by adjusting population and mortality for differential underestimation using the National Mortality Follow-back Survey [1,31]. Following Hahn and Eberhardt [1], age- and sex-specific correction factors were applied to population and mortality figures for Asians (America 1), with the excess mortality or population coming from Middle America (America 3), the group to which Asians are most likely to be misclassified.

Data Sources on Health Plan Coverage and Health-Care Utilization

Data on health plan coverage and health-care utilization were from the Behavioral Risk Factor Surveillance System (BRFSS). The BRFSS is an annual cross-sectional telephone survey conducted by the Centers for Disease Control and Prevention and state health departments. The BRFSS uses a multistage cluster design based on random-digit dialing to select a representative sample from each state's noninstitutionalized civilian residents aged 18 y and older, and is described in detail elsewhere [32,33] and in online documentation (http://www.cdc.gov/brfss). The BRFSS questionnaire primarily focuses on personal risk behaviors and exposures, but also includes questions on health plan coverage and utilization of care. The

BRFSS data for 2001–2003 were averaged to reduce sensitivity to interannual fluctuations. Counties were matched to the appropriate America using the standardized Federal Information Processing Standards (FIPS) county codes. Counties with unidentifiable codes (<1% of all counties) were excluded from the analysis. The BRFSS survey instrument on health-care access asks about health-care coverage status including health insurance, prepaid plans such as HMOs, and government programs such as Medicare or Medicaid. The BRFSS also asks about time since the last routine checkup. BRFSS data from the latest 2–3 y before the analysis were used: 2001–2003 for health-care coverage and 2001–2002 for checkup (this variable was not included in the 2003 BRFSS).

Data for International Comparisons

Data on life expectancy and probabilities of death (all-cause and disease-specific) for international comparisons were from the Global Burden of Disease databases, maintained by the World Health Organization [34,35].

Analysis Methods

Period all-cause and cause-eliminated life expectancies and probabilities of death were calculated using standard demographic life-table techniques [36].

RESULTS

Definition of the Eight Americas

Table 1 summarizes the characteristics of the eight Americas (see also Figures S1 and S2). America 1 consists of Asians, excluding those living in counties where Pacific Islanders make up more than 40% of the total Asian population. Asians in the latter group of counties were included in America 3. The 10.1 million Asians in America 1 have levels income and education almost exactly even with the national average. America 2 consists of northland (Minnesota, the Dakotas, Iowa, Montana, and Nebraska) low-income rural white populations, with income and education below the national average. America 3 is Middle America, the large fraction of the US population that has slightly above-average per capita income and education. This group largely consists of white Americans (98% of America 3), but also includes small numbers of Asians and Native Americans living in counties that are not included in Americas 1 and 5. America 4 consists of low-income white populations in Appalachia and the Mississippi Valley,

30% of whom have not completed high school. America 5 is made up of Native Americans living in the West, excluding the West Coast. The majority of this group lives on or near reservations, mostly in the Four Corners region (where the borders of Arizona, Colorado, New Mexico, and Utah meet) or the Dakotas. America 7 comprises low-income rural blacks in the Mississippi Valley and the Deep South. America 8 includes blacks living in high-risk urban environments. America 6 represents the rest of black America, living mostly in urban or semi-urban counties.

Mortality Experiences of the Eight Americas

Figure 3 summarizes the mortality experiences for the eight Americas between 1982 and 2001, divided into broad age groups and diseases in Figure 4A for 2001. Asian Americans have sustained extraordinary advantage over the nearest groups, the northland low-income white rural populations (America 2; 5.9 y higher life expectancy for males and 5.6 y for females in 2001; 5.5 and 7.3 y, respectively, in 1982) and Middle America (America 3; 6.8 y higher life expectancy for males and 7.1 y for females in 2001; 6.8 and 9.3 y, respectively, in 1982). Therefore, although many second-generation (US-born) Asians have entered the adult cohorts, the sustained gap between America 1 and other groups has not narrowed over the last 20 y (see also Singh and Miller [4]).

The gap between the life expectancy of the 3.4 million black males in high-risk urban areas in America 8 and the life expectancy for the 5.5 million Asian females in America 1 in 2001 was 20.7 y. Within the sexes, the gap between the best-off and the worst-off groups was 15.4 y for males (Asians versus blacks in high-risk urban areas) and 12.8 y for females (Asians versus low-income southern rural blacks). These gaps are 2.4 and 2.8 times those between white and black life expectancies for the nation as a whole for males and females, respectively. During the late 1980s and early 1990s, the gap between Americas 1 and 8 for males widened significantly, mostly because of higher HIV and homicide death rates. Excluding this period, the gap in male life expectancy between Americas 1 and 8 increased by half a year between 1982 and 2001. Excluding the first few years of the 1980s, when there was an unexplained decline in life expectancy of Asian females, the gap in female life expectancy between Americas 1 and 8 declined by 2.5 y; the gap in life expectancy between Asian females and low-income southern rural black females (America 7) decreased by 1 y (from 13.8 to 12.8 y).

The 12.8-y gap in life expectancy between females in Americas 1 and 7 is approximately the same as the gap between Japan, with the highest national life expectancy for females in 2001 (84.7 y), and Fiji, Nicaragua, and Lebanon [34]. Asian females in the US have a life expectancy that is

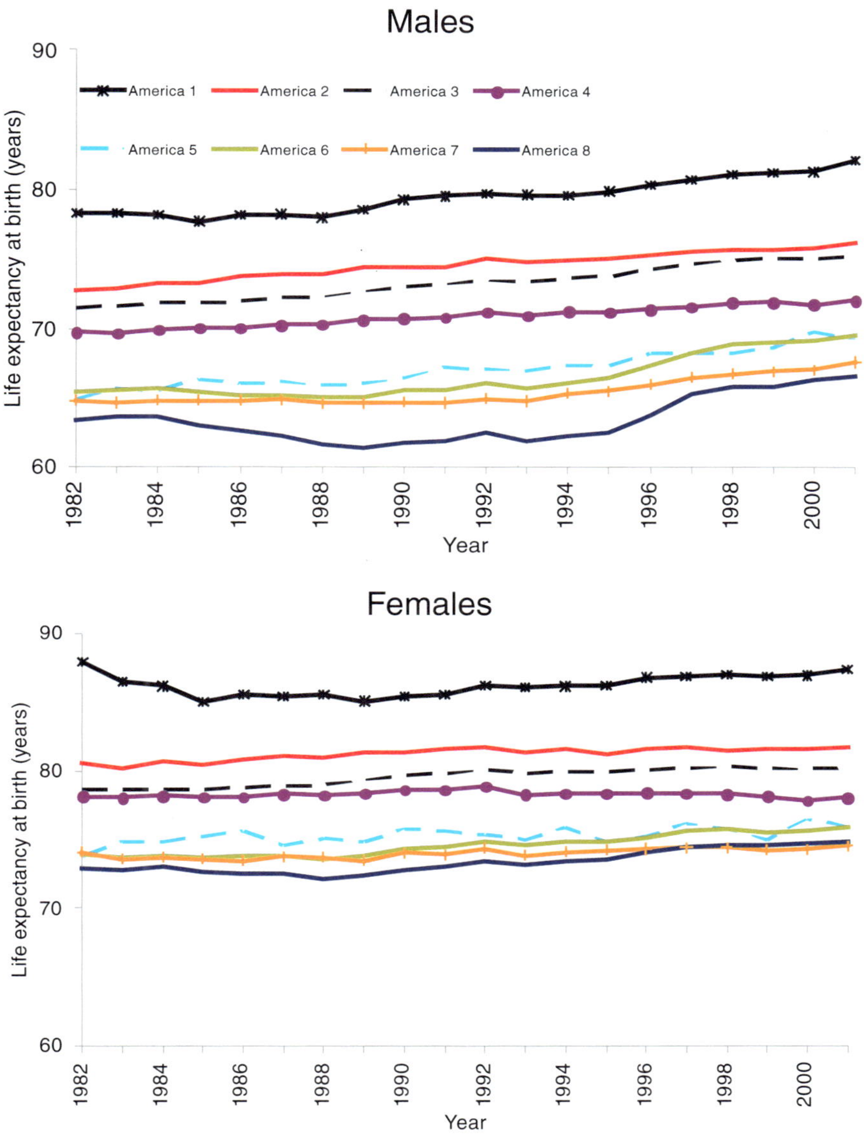

Figure 3. Life Expectancy at Birth in the Eight Americas (1982–2001)
Estimates for Americas 1 and 3 have been adjusted for differential underestimation of population and mortality among Asians (see Methods).
DOI: 10.1371/journal.pmed.0030260.g003

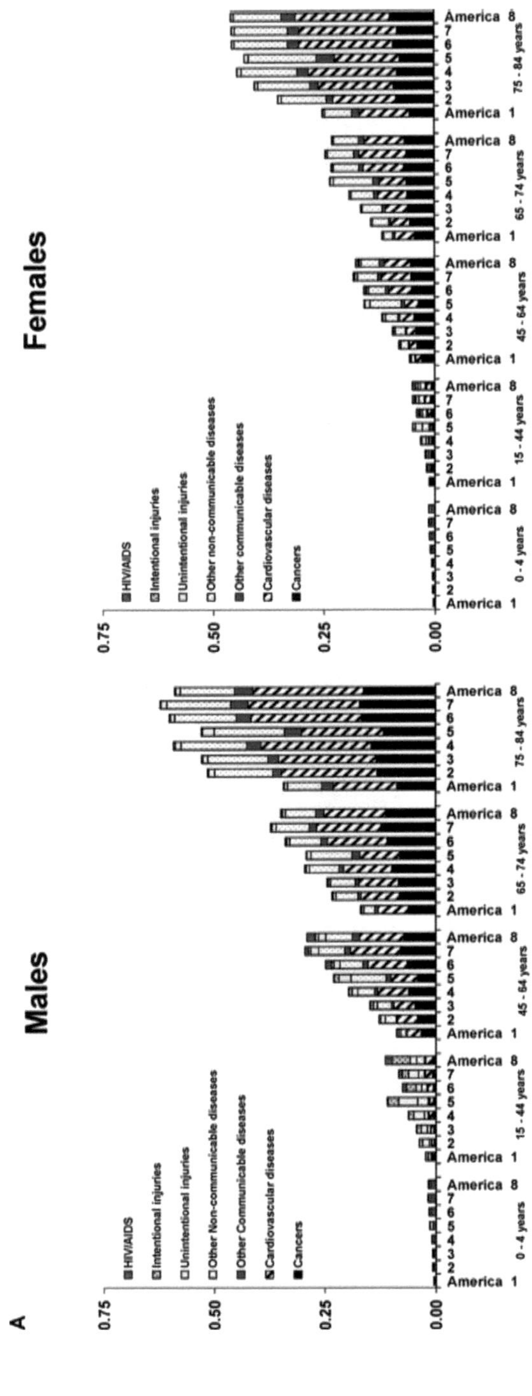
A
Males
Females
0.75
0.50
0.25
0.00
HIV/AIDS
Intentional injuries
Unintentional injuries
Other Non-communicable diseases
Other Communicable diseases
Cardiovascular diseases
Cancers
Other non-communicable diseases
Other communicable diseases
America 1
2
3
4
5
6
7
America 8
0 - 4 years
15 - 44 years
45 - 64 years
65 - 74 years
75 - 84 years

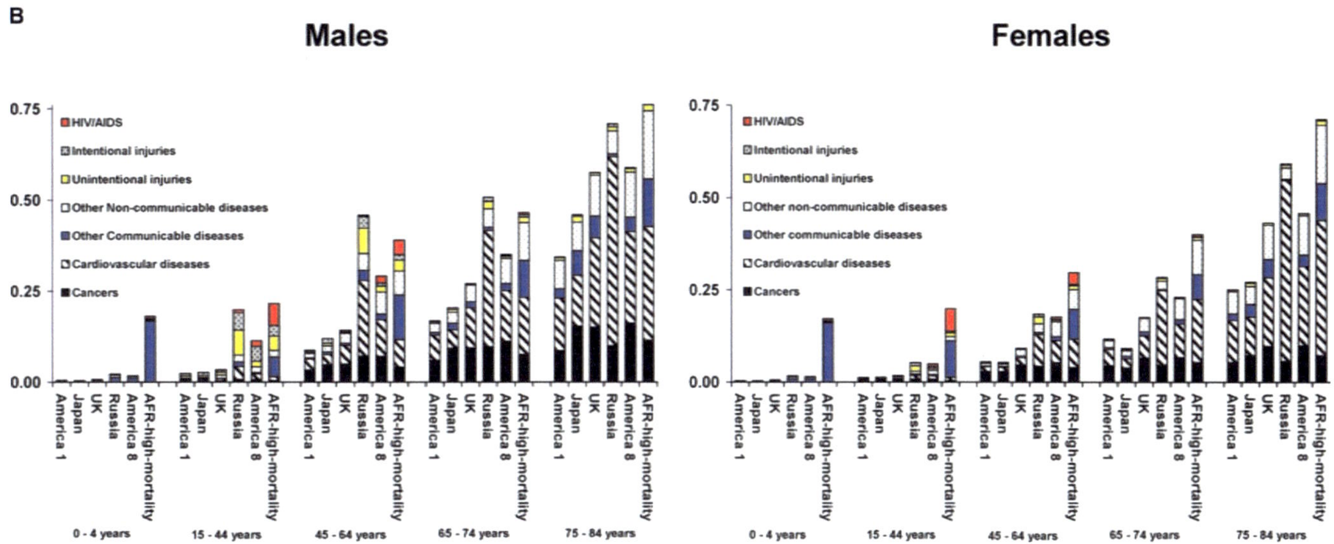

Figure 4. Probability of Dying in Specific Age Ranges in the Eight Americas

(A) Probability of death by sex, age, and disease for the eight Americas in 2001.

(B) Probability of death by sex, age, and disease for Americas 1 and 8 compared to Japan, UK, the Russian Federation, and high-mortality countries in sub-Saharan Africa (AFR-high-mortality; made up largely of countries in West Africa and excluding countries with very high mortality due to HIV/AIDS) in 2001.

Results are not shown for ages 5–14 y because there are few deaths in this age range in the US.

DOI: 10.1371/journal.pmed.0030260.g004

3 y higher than that of females in Japan [34]. For males, the 15.4-y gap in life expectancy between Asians (America 1) and high-risk urban blacks (America 8) is the same as between Iceland, with the highest national male life expectancy in 2001 (78.2 y), and Sao Tome, Belarus, and Uzbekistan [34]. In other words, millions of Americans, distinctly identified by their sociodemographic characteristics and place of residence, have life expectancies that are similar to some low-income developing countries (see also Figure 4B).

The eight Americas classification reveals that within the white population there is a wide variation in health experience that cannot be explained by differences in average income: low-income white rural populations in Minnesota, the Dakotas, Iowa, Montana, and Nebraska (America 2), with a life expectancy of 76.2 and 81.8 y for males and females, respectively, have a substantial advantage over the rest of white America, despite a large income disadvantage. Low-income whites in Appalachia and the Mississippi Valley (America 4), with an average income level similar to that of America 2, have a life expectancy equal to those of Mexico and Panama. The life expectancy gap between whites in America 2 and America 4 was 4.2 and 3.8 y in 2001 for males and females, respectively, comparable to the 6.4- and 4.6-y gaps between whites and blacks as a whole. The gap between whites in America 2 and America 4 has in fact increased since 1982, when it was 3.0 and 2.4 y for males and females respectively; between 1982 and 2001 life expectancy among females in America 4 declined from 78.2 y to 78.1 y.

Because America 3 is the largest subgroup of the US population, we investigated the potential role of sociodemographic and geographical predictors used to define the eight Americas in morality patterns within America 3. County-level analysis of mortality for 1997–2001 shows that average life expectancy for whites in America 3 (98% of America 3 are whites) was 77.1 y, with a standard deviation of 1.7 y. The correlation coefficient between county-level life expectancy and per capita income in 2000 was 0.35. Life expectancy ranged from 76.7 to 78.3 y in the quartiles of county-level per capita income; it ranged from 77.0 to 78.6 y in quartiles of county-level education (based on proportion who have completed high school). The highest county-level education quartile consistently had the highest life expectancy over time, but there was no consistent education gradient for the other three quartiles. There was also no obvious geographical pattern in mortality in America 3 (Figure 1). For example, life expectancy for counties east and west of the Mississippi River was 76.6 and 77.2 y, respectively.

Although at the national level Native Americans seemingly had a life expectancy equal to or higher than whites, Native Americans living in the West, mostly on or near reservations (America 5) and with the lowest per capita income of all the eight Americas had a major mortality disadvantage. Life expectancies for America 5 were 5.9 and 4.3 y lower than Middle America (America 3) for males and females, respectively, in 2001. Cause-of-death analysis for America 5 demonstrates that this Native American population has very high rates of mortality from alcohol-related causes such as road traffic accidents and cirrhosis of the liver, as well as diabetes (Figure 4A). Across the three black Americas (black Middle America, southern low-income rural, and high-risk urban), the gap in life expectancy in 2001 was 1 y for females and nearly 3 y for males. The male gap was as wide as 4 y in the mid-1990s, with the subsequent decline mostly due to reduction in HIV/AIDS mortality.

Age and Disease Patterns of Mortality in the Eight Americas

Figure 4 shows mortality risk in four age groups (0–4, 15–44, 45–64, and 65–74 y) for the eight Americas, and further compares Americas 1 and 8 with countries and regions at a range of mortality levels including Japan, the United Kingdom, the Russian Federation, and the high-mortality countries of sub-Saharan Africa. Although an imporant gradient in child mortality remains between America 1 and America 8, a disadvantaged child in the US has an order of magnitude lower risk of death compared to low-income nations in sub-Saharan Africa. Above 70 y of age, disparities in mortality in the eight Americas are also reduced, especially in international comparisons. This pattern is partly because of the generally higher mortality in this age group and possibly also because of cohort effects.

The mortality disparities in the eight Americas are largest for young (ages 15–44) and middle-aged adults (ages 45–64). In these age groups, blacks living in high-risk urban areas (America 8) have mortality risks more similar to ones in the Russian Federation and sub-Saharan Africa, which are substantially higher than those in America 1, Japan, or the United Kingdom. In 2001, 15-y-old black men and women in high-risk urban areas (America 8) were, respectively, 3.8 and 3.4 times as likely as those in America 1 to die before the age of 60 (Figure 5A), and 4.7 and 3.8 times more likely before the age of 45. The disparity in young and middle-aged adult mortality between America 8 and America 1 has increased since 1982, when the mortality risk ratio was 3.4 and 2.8 for men and women, respectively. The excess young and middle-aged mortality persists after removing the effects of HIV and homicide (Figure 5B). Rather, the major mortality gradients in these age groups are observed for injuries, cardiovascular diseases, and other noncommunicable causes such as liver cirrhosis and diabetes (Figure 4A). Injuries are especially important for the observed mortality gradients between the ages of 15 and 44.

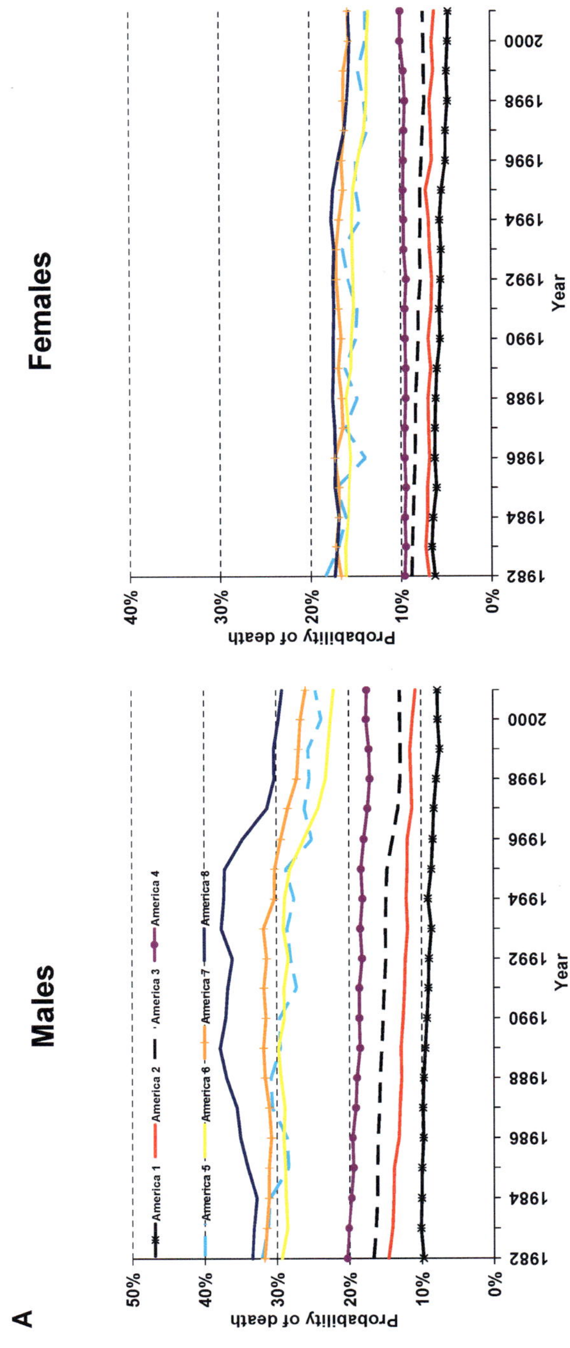
A
Males
Females
America 1
America 2
America 3
America 4
America 5
America 6
America 7
America 8
Probability of death
50%
40%
30%
20%
10%
0%
Year
1982
1984
1986
1988
1990
1992
1994
1996
1998
2000

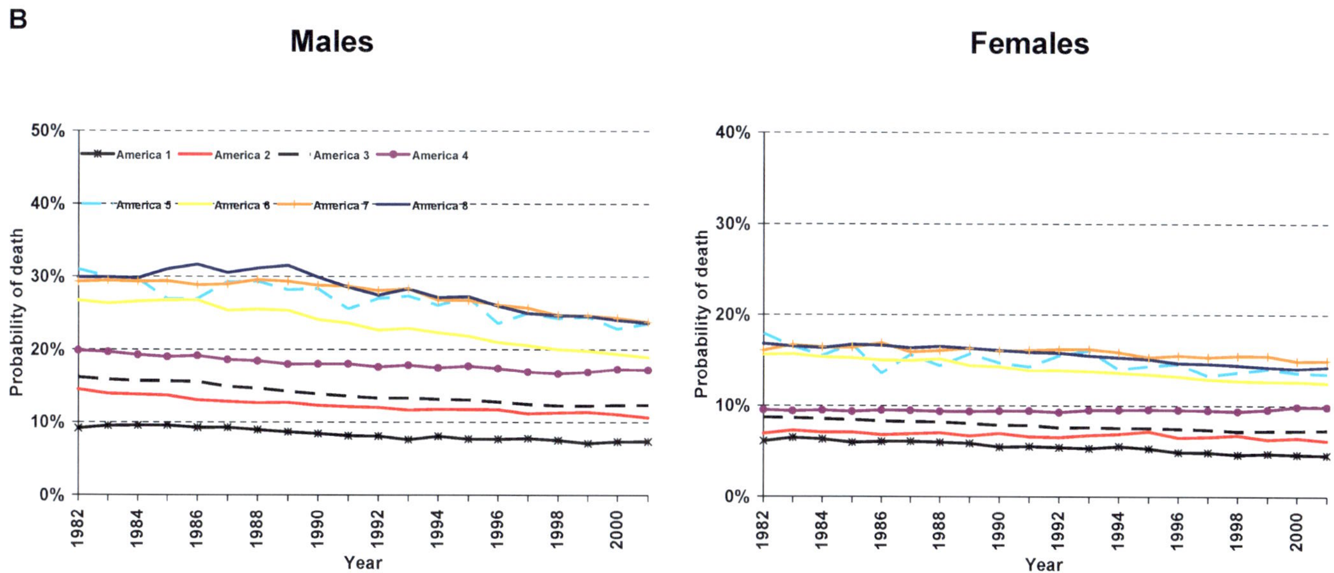

Figure 5. Probability of Death between the Ages of 15 and 59 y in the Eight Americas
(A) Probability of death between the ages of 15 and 59 y in the eight Americas from all causes.
(B) Probability of death between the ages of 15 and 59 y in the eight Americas after deleting deaths from homicide and HIV.
DOI: 10.1371/journal.pmed.0030260.g005

Health-Care Access and Utilization

Figure 6A shows self-reported health plan coverage in the eight Americas. Native Americans in the West (America 5) reported the lowest coverage, followed by low-income rural southern blacks (America 7). The highest coverage was in northland white low-income rural populations (America 2), followed by Middle America and Asians (Americas 3 and 1). Basic health system encounter, measured as the fraction reporting a routine checkup in the past 12 mo, also shows relatively small variation across the eight Americas. For both males and females, the rates of routine checkup are slightly higher in Americas 6, 7, and 8, the groups with mortality disadvantage.

DISCUSSION

The eight Americas in this paper consist of distinct subgroups of the US population defined based on a small number of sociodemographic and geographical indicators including race, the location of the county of residence, population density, race-specific county-level per capita income, and cumulative homicide rate. Put in a global context, the disparities in mortality experiences among the eight Americas, each consisting of millions or tens of millions of Americans, are enormous. The eight Americas analysis indicates that ten million Americans with the best health have achieved one of the highest levels of life expectancy on record, 3 y better than Japan for females and 4 y better than Iceland for males. At the same time, tens of millions of Americans are experiencing levels of health that are more typical of middle-income or low-income developing countries. These poor levels of

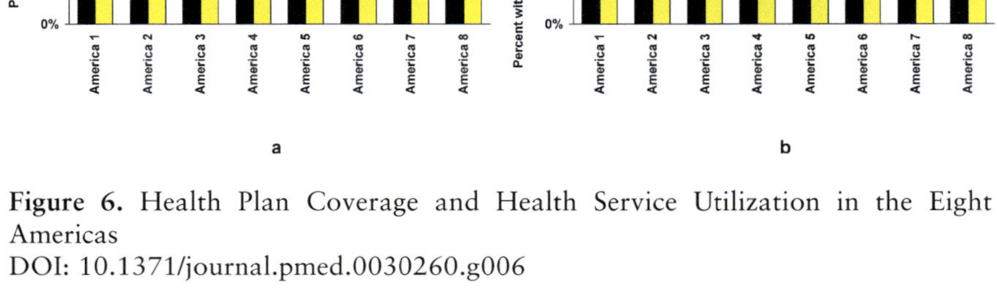

Figure 6. Health Plan Coverage and Health Service Utilization in the Eight Americas
DOI: 10.1371/journal.pmed.0030260.g006

health occur in areas throughout the country. The health disparities among the eight Americas cannot be explained by single causes of death such as homicide or HIV. Nor are the largest sources of disparity in children and the elderly. The mortality disparities are most concentrated in young and middle-aged males and females, and are a result of a number of chronic diseases and injuries with well-established risk factors.

Trends in life expectancy show that neither the relative ordering nor the absolute levels of life expectancy disparities among the eight Americas decreased between 1982 and 2001. During the late 1980s and early 1990s, the life expectancy gap between America 8 and the remaining groups widened significantly for males, mostly because of HIV and homicide rates. In this overall picture of stable disparities, there have been specific groups whose mortality has worsened. For example, the life expectancy of low-income white females in Appalachia and the Mississippi Valley declined between 1982 and 2001.

The most important limitation of the data used for our analysis is that reported race in the census, used for population estimates, may be different from race in mortality statistics, where race may be reported by the family, the certifying physician, or the funeral director [1,31]. Sensitivity to differential race reporting would be largest for those groups with small population and a relatively large proportion of mixed-race individuals, mainly the Native Americans and Asians [1,31]. In these groups, it is more likely for race to be reported as Native American or Asian in the census than it is in the death certificate; hence, the differential underestimation of deaths and population results in bias in the form of a net underestimation of mortality [1,31]. The mortality and population for Asians were corrected for differential underestimation, using the National Mortality Followback Survey [1,31] (Correction using the National Longitudinal Mortality Study would have given virtually identical estimates: 12% underreporting of mortality in the National Mortality Followback Survey versus 13% in the National Longitudinal Mortality Study [31]). For Native Americans, misreporting race on death certificates is most important where mixed races exist and Native Americans form a small proportion of the population (e.g., in California). The grouping used in the eight Americas distinguished between those Native Americans who primarily live on or near reservations (America 5) and the remaining Native Americans (included in America 3), and is therefore robust to this error because living on or near reservations increases the likelihood of correct race recording on death certificates. Any residual bias would be in the form of net underestimation of mortality as described above and as observed nationally for Native Americans [31]. Mortality underestimation would in turn imply that life expectancy is even lower in America 5, and hence further magnify the findings of the above analysis on mortality disadvantage in America 5.

A secondary source of bias for Asians may be back-migration of first-generation immigrants, who return to their home countries due to illness. This would lead to an underreporting of deaths for Asians, and overestimation of life expectancy in America 1. To examine the effect of this source of bias, we repeated the analysis restricting the sample to US-born Asians. Excluding the two states (Alaska and Hawaii) whose Asian population is entirely in America 3 (and not in America 1), US-born Asian females and males had life expectancies at birth that were, respectively, 5.1 and 1.6 y higher than those for combined US-born and foreign-born Asians together, consistent with previous findings on immigrant populations [4]. Lower mortality in US-born Asians confirms that the patterns in Figures 3–5 are not a result of unrecorded mortality due to return migration among Asian populations; rather, they represent a real mortality advantage in America 1.

The findings on persistent health disparities in the eight Americas raise the question of why, as a society, we have failed to narrow health gaps between distinct and large subgroups of the US population. Opportunities and interventions to reduce health inequalities include (1) reducing socioeconomic inequalities, which are the distal causes of health inequalities, (2) increasing financial access to health care by decreasing the number of Americans without health plan coverage, (3) removing physical, behavioral, and cultural barriers to health care, (4) reducing disparities in the quality of care, (5) designing public health strategies and interventions to reduce health risks at the level of communities (e.g., changes in urban/neighborhood design to facilitate physical activity and reduce obesity), and (6) designing public health strategies to reduce health risks that target individuals or population subgroups that are not necessarily in the same community (e.g., tobacco taxation or pharmacological interventions for blood pressure and cholesterol).

Important research in the past few decades has illustrated the critical role of individual and community-level socioeconomic factors, be it in absolute or relative terms, in health outcomes [11,24,37,38]. In addition to (or in the absence of, as is currently the case in the US) systematic policies for reducing socioeconomic inequalities, public health and health care provide instruments for addressing inequalities in health outcomes. Much of the health policy agenda in the US is currently focused on health insurance coverage for the nearly 44 million Americans (15% of the population) who lack health insurance [39,40]. Although increasing insurance coverage and access to care would most likely contribute to narrowing disparities across the eight Americas, the available data (Figure 6) suggest that the variation in health plan coverage across the eight Americas is small relative to the very large gradient in health outcomes. It is likely that expanding insurance coverage alone would still leave huge disparities in young and middle-aged adults. A shortcoming of the BRFSS data on health insurance and health-care utilization, however, is that they do not provide any insight into the likely contribution of variation in quality of care to the disparities across the eight Americas.

The diseases with the largest contribution to mortality disparities across the eight Americas are chronic diseases and injuries with well-established risk factors, including alcohol use, tobacco smoking, overweight and obesity, and elevated blood pressure, cholesterol, and glucose. These risk factors are also the leading cause of burden of disease in the nation as a whole (Figure 7). An important question, therefore, is the distributions of exposure to these risks in the eight Americas, and the fraction of disease-specific and all-cause mortality attributable to their hazardous effects. This is particularly relevant for combinations of risk factors that together account for large proportions of many chronic diseases [41,42]. Definite estimates of the contributions of risk factors to health inequalities require analyses for race-county combinations, which are not readily possible using currently available data: among data sources on risk factors, the BRFSS allows subnational analysis but relies on self-reported exposure. Although self-reported exposure is the common metric for risks such as tobacco smoking and alcohol use, it is subject to bias for overweight and obesity and for elevated blood pressure, cholesterol, and glucose because of individual reporting behavior and because individuals may not be aware of their blood pressure, cholesterol, and glucose status. The National Health and Nutrition Examination Survey provides measurements of this latter group of risks, but does not include sufficient geographical detail for analysis at the county or even state level [25]. Methods for combining the two data sources to obtain estimates for population subgroups based on race and place of residence are required [43]. If analysis of risk factors illustrates that a substantial proportion of disparities among the eight Americas are attributable to risk factor exposure, risk factor interventions should be investigated as tools for reducing health inequalities, in the same way that they have been used for achieving aggregate national health benefits. The interventions will likely include both population-wide measures (e.g., tobacco taxation, drinking-and-driving countermeasures, and interventions to reduce public and domestic alcohol-induced violence) and personal interventions (e.g., pharmacological interventions for blood pressure and cholesterol).

The traditional emphasis of the US health system has been on children and the elderly, as, for example, illustrated by the low levels of resources devoted to injury prevention and tobacco control compared with immunization [44]. This emphasis may have partly contributed to substantially lower disparities in these age groups relative to young and middle-aged adults. On the other hand, the emphasis on children and the elderly has treated many of the diseases that are important contributors to young

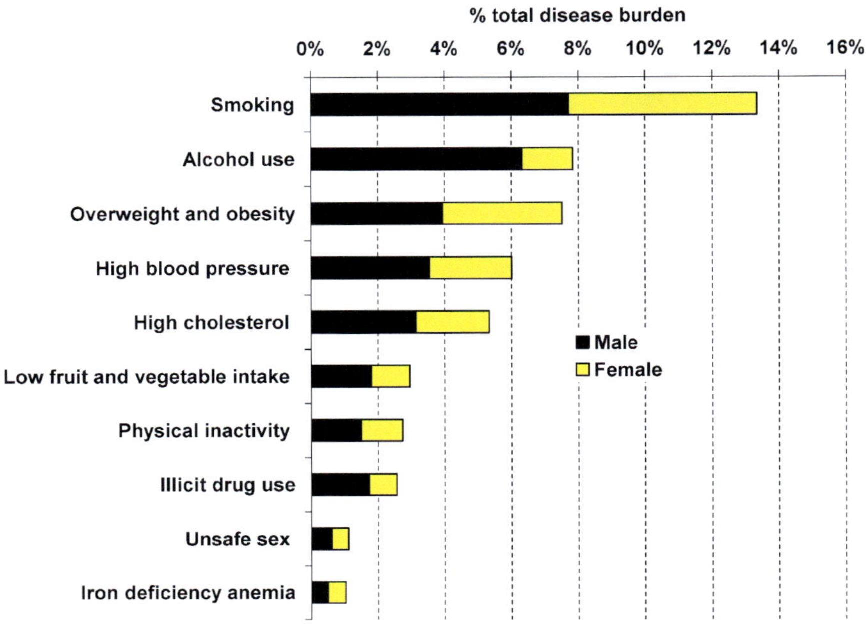

Figure 7. Burden of Disease Attributable to the Ten Leading Risk Factors in the very-low-mortality countries of the Region of Americas
The estimates refer to the Global Burden of Disease epidemiological region that includes Canada, Cuba, and the US [45]; more than 85% of this region's population live in the US and most data sources apply to the US.
DOI: 10.1371/journal.pmed.0030260.g007

and middle-aged adult health disparities, and their risk factors, as either the responsibilities of individuals (alcohol, tobacco, obesity, and dietary determinants of blood pressure and cholesterol, like salt) or in the domain of clinical care (blood pressure and cholesterol). A number of important steps are needed to broaden the current perspective. First, there is a need to use systematic epidemiological and economic analyses to identify effective and cost-effective health interventions—whether targeting populations or individuals—that would make the biggest difference to those with the worst health. Given the distinct epidemiological, geographical, and sociodemographic profiles of the eight Americas, the leading interventions may be different for each, although some common core strategies may exist (e.g., common core cardiovascular disease prevention strategies). Second, monitoring systems should be developed by the states and territories to provide local but benchmarked information on the fraction of the population in each community who would benefit from these interventions and are receiving them. Third, information on the delivery of these interventions for different communities should be publicly reported. It is when the public, community and professional groups, media, and politicians focus attention on what is being achieved, and why efforts are working in some places and not others, that the culture of accountability for health outcomes will be strengthened.

SUPPORTING INFORMATION

Dataset S1. Life Expectancy at Birth by County
Found at 10.1371/journal.pmed.0030260.sd001 (4 MB XLS).
Figure S1. Geographic Locations for Americas 2, 3, and 4
Found at 10.1371/journal.pmed.0030260.sg001 (549 KB PDF).
Figure S2. Geographic Locations for Americas 6, 7, and 8
Found at 10.1371/journal.pmed.0030260.sg002 (268 KB PDF).

ACKNOWLEDGMENTS

We thank J. Holt, J. Marks, M. McKenna, G. Mensah, and J. Salomon for valuable discussions and comments.

Author contributions. CJLM and ME designed the study. SCK, CM, NT, MTB, and TJI analyzed data and constructed figures and maps. CJLM, SCK, and ME wrote the paper.

REFERENCES

1. Hahn RA, Eberhardt S (1995) Life expectancy in four U.S. racial/ethnic populations: 1990. Epidemiology 6: 350–355.
2. Wong MD, Shapiro MF, Boscardin WJ, Ettner SL (2002) Contribution of major diseases to disparities in mortality. N Engl J Med 347: 1585–1592.
3. Singh GK, Yu SM (1996) Trends and differentials in adolescent and young adult mortality in the United States, 1950 through 1993. Am J Public Health 86: 560–564.
4. Singh GK, Miller BA (2004) Health, life expectancy, and mortality patterns among immigrant populations in the United States. Can J Public Health 95: 14–21.
5. Cooper R, Cutler J, Desvigne-Nickens P, Fortmann S, Friedman L, et al. (2000) Trends and disparities in coronary heart disease, stroke, and other cardiovascular diseases in the United States: Findings of the national conference on cardiovascular disease prevention. Circulation 102: 3137–3147.
6. Navarro V (1990) Race or class versus race and class: Mortality differentials in the United States. Lancet 336: 1238–1240.
7. Geronimus AT, Bound J, Waidmann TA, Hillemeier MM, Burns PB (1996) Excess mortality among blacks and whites in the United States. N Engl J Med 335: 1552–1558.

8. Geronimus AT, Bound J, Waidmann TA (1999) Poverty, time, and place: Variation in excess mortality across selected US populations, 1980–1990. J Epidemiol Community Health 53: 325–334.
9. Hahn RA, Eaker ED, Barker ND, Teutsch SM, Sosniak WA, et al. (1996) Poverty and death in the United States. Int J Health Serv 26: 673–690.
10. Isaacs SL, Schroeder SA (2004) Class—The ignored determinant of the nation's health. N Engl J Med 351: 1137–1142.
11. Adler N, Marmot M, McEwan B, Stewart J, editors (1999) Socioeconomic status and health in industrial nations: Social, psychological, and biological pathways. New York: New York Academy of Science. 503 p.
12. Singh GK (2003) Area deprivation and widening inequalities in US mortality, 1969–1998. Am J Public Health 93: 1137–1143.
13. Muntaner C, Eaton WW, Miech R, O'Campo P (2004) Socioeconomic position and major mental disorders. Epidemiol Rev 26: 53–62.
14. Pappas G, Queen S, Hadden W, Fisher G (1993) The increasing disparity in mortality between socioeconomic groups in the United States, 1960 and 1986. N Engl J Med 329: 103–109.
15. Davey Smith G, Neaton JD, Wentworth D, Stamler R, Stamler J (1998) Mortality differences between black and white men in the USA: Contribution of income and other risk factors among men screened for the MRFIT. MRFIT Research Group. Multiple Risk Factor Intervention Trial. Lancet 351: 934–939.
16. Krieger N, Chen JT, Waterman PD, Rehkopf DH, Subramanian SV (2005) Painting a truer picture of US socioeconomic and racial/ethnic health inequalities: The Public Health Disparities Geocoding Project. Am J Public Health 95: 312–323.
17. Smedley BD, Stith AY, Nelson AR, editors (2003) Unequal treatment: Confronting racial and ethnic disparities in health care. Washington (D.C.): National Academy Press. 764 p.
18. Bloche MG (2004) Health care disparities—Science, politics, and race. N Engl J Med 350: 1568–1570.
19. Gornick ME, Eggers PW, Riley GF (2001) Understanding disparities in the use of Medicare services. Yale J Health Policy Law Ethics 1: 133–158.
20. Gornick ME, Eggers PW, Reilly TW, Mentnech RM, Fitterman LK, et al. (1996) Effects of race and income on mortality and use of services among Medicare beneficiaries. N Engl J Med 335: 791–799.
21. Epstein AM, Ayanian JZ (2001) Racial disparities in medical care. N Engl J Med 344: 1471–1473.
22. Goldman DP, Smith JP (2002) Can patient self-management help explain the SES health gradient? Proc Natl Acad Sci U S A 99: 10929–10934.
23. Murray CJL, Michaud C, Mckenna MT, Marks JS (1998) US patterns of mortality by county and race: 1965–1994. Atlanta and Boston: Centers for Disease Control and Prevention and Harvard Center for Population and Development Studies. Available: http://www.hsph.harvard.edu/organizations/bdu/images/usbodi/index.html. Accessed 11 July 2006.
24. Mackenbach JP, Bakker MJ (2003) Tackling socioeconomic inequalities in health: Analysis of European experiences. Lancet 362: 1409–1414.
25. Otten MW Jr, Teutsch SM, Williamson DF, Marks JS (1990) The effect of known risk factors on the excess mortality of black adults in the United States. JAMA 263: 845–850.
26. Stafford M, Bartley M, Mitchell R, Marmot M (2001) Characteristics of individuals and characteristics of areas: Investigating their influence on health in the Whitehall II study. Health Place 7: 117–129.

27. Stafford M, Marmot M (2003) Neighbourhood deprivation and health: Does it affect us all equally? Int J Epidemiol 32: 357–366.
28. Ingram DD, Parker JD, Schenker N, Weed JA, Hamilton B, et al. (2003) United States Census 2000 population with bridged race categories. Vital Health Stat 2: 1–55.
29. US Census Bureau. 1990 Census Summary Tape File 3. Available: http://factfinder.census.gov/servlet/DatasetMainPageServlet?_program¼DEC&_tabId¼DEC2&_submenuId¼datasets_1&_lang¼en&_ts¼171635619510. Accessed 25 July 2006.
30. National Center for Health Statistics (2006) Mortality data, multiple cause-of-death public-use data files. Hyattsville (Maryland): National Center for Health Statistics. Available: http://www.cdc.gov/nchs/products/elec_prods/subject/mortmcd.htm Accessed 13 July 2006.
31. Rosenberg H, Maurer J, Sorlie P, Johnson N, MacDorman MF, et al. (1999) Quality of death rates by race and Hispanic origin: A summary of current research, 1999. Vital Health Stat 2: 1–13.
32. Nelson DE, Holtzman D, Waller M, Leutzinger CL, Condon K (1998) Objectives and design of the Behavioral Risk Factor Surveillance System. In: Proceedings of the Survey Research Methods Section, American Statistical Association National Meeting (1998). Alexandria (Virginia): American Statistical Association. Available: http://www.amstat.org/sections/srms/proceedings/papers/1998_032.pdf. Accessed 11 July 2006.
33. Remington PL, Smith MY, Williamson DF, Anda RF, Gentry EM, et al. (1988) Design, characteristics, and usefulness of state-based behavioral risk factor surveillance: 1981–87. Public Health Rep 103: 366–375.
34. World Health Organization (2002) The world health report 2002: Reducing risks, promoting healthy life. Geneva: World Health Organization. Available: http://www.who.int/whr/2002/en/whr02_en.pdf. Accessed 11 July 2006.
35. Mathers CD, Lopez AD, Murray CJL (2006) The burden of disease and mortality by condition: Data, methods, and results for 2001. In: Lopez AD, Mathers CD, Ezzati M, Jamison DT, Murray CJL, editors. Global burden of disease and risk factors. New York: Oxford University Press. pp. 45–240. Available: http://files.dcp2.org/pdf/GBD/GBD03.pdf. Accessed 21 July 2006.
36. Preston SH, Heuveline P, Guillot M (2001) Demography: Measuring and modeling population processes. Oxford: Blackwell Publishing. 291 p.
37. Marmot MG (2003) Understanding social inequalities in health. Perspect Biol Med 46: 9–23.
38. Marmot M (2002) The influence of income on health: Views of an epidemiologist. Does money really matter? Or is it a marker for something else? Health Aff (Millwood) 21: 31–46.
39. US Census Bureau (2003) Health insurance coverage in the United States: 2002. Washington (D.C.): US Census Bureau. Available: http://www.census.gov/prod/2003pubs/p60–223.pdf. Accessed 21 July 2006.
40. McCanne DR (2004) A national health insurance program for the United States. PLoS Medicine 1: e39. DOI: 10.1371/journal.pmed.0010039.
41. Ezzati M, Vander Hoorn S, Rodgers A, Lopez AD, Mathers CD, et al. (2003) Estimates of global and regional potential health gains from reducing multiple major risk factors. Lancet 362: 271–280.
42. Yusuf S, Hawken S, Ounpuu S, Dans T, Avezum A, et al. (2004) Effect of potentially modifiable risk factors associated with myocardial infarction in 52 countries (the INTERHEART study): Case-control study. Lancet 364: 937–952.
43. Ezzati M, Martin H, Skjold S, Vander HS, Murray CJL (2006) Trends in national and state-level obesity in the USA after correction for self-report bias: Analysis of health surveys. J R Soc Med 99: 250–257.

44. Centers for Disease Control and Prevention (2005) FY 2005 CDC appropriation—Budget by functional area. Available: http://www.cdc.gov/fmo/PDFs/FY05FundFunctAreaTable.pdf. Accessed 21 July 2006.
45. Ezzati M, Lopez AD, Rodgers A, Vander Hoorn S, Murray CJL, et al. (2002) Selected major risk factors and global and regional burden of disease. Lancet 360: 1347–1360.

EDITORS' SUMMARY

Background

It has been recognized for a long time that the number of years that people in the United States can expect to live ("life expectancy") varies enormously. For example, white Americans tend to live longer than black Americans, and life expectancy is much greater in some of the roughly 3,000 counties of the US than it is in others. However, there is a lack of information and understanding on how big a part is played in "health inequalities" by specific diseases and injuries, by risk factors (such as tobacco, alcohol, and obesity), and by variations in access to effective health care.

Why Was This Study Done?

The researchers wanted to find a way of dividing the people of the US into groups based on a small number of characteristics—such as location of county of residence, race, and income—that would help demonstrate the most important factors accounting for differences in life expectancy.

What Did the Researchers Do and Find?

The researchers used figures from the US Census Bureau and the National Center for Health Statistics to calculate mortality (death) rates for the years 1982–2001. They took note of the county of residence and of the race of all the people who died during that period of time. This enabled them to calculate the mortality rates for all 8,221 "race-county units" (all of the individuals of a given race in a given county). They experimented with different ways of combining the race-counties into a small and manageable number of groups. They eventually settled on the idea of there being "eight Americas," defined on the basis of race-county, population density, income, and homicide rate. Each group contains millions or tens of millions of people. For each of the eight groups the researchers estimated life expectancy, the risk of mortality from specific diseases, the proportion of people who had health insurance, and people's routine encounters with health-care services. (The researchers also created maps of life expectancies for the US counties.) They describe their eight Americas as follows: Asians, northland low-income rural whites, Middle America, low-income whites in Appalachia and the Mississippi Valley, western Native Americans, black Middle America, low-income southern rural blacks, and high-risk urban blacks.

Many striking differences in life expectancy were found between the eight groups. For example, in 2001, the life expectancy gap between the 3.4 million high-risk urban black males and the 5.6 million Asian females was nearly 21 years. Within the sexes, the life expectancy gap between the best-off and the worst-off groups was 15.4 years for males (Asians versus high-risk urban blacks) and 12.8 years for females (Asians versus low-income rural blacks in the South). The causes of death that were mainly responsible for these variations were various chronic diseases and injury. The gaps between best-off and worst-off were similar in 2001 to what they were in 1987.

What Do These Findings Mean?

Health inequalities in the US are large and are showing no sign of reducing. Social and economic reforms would certainly help change the situation. At the same time, the public health system should also improve the way in which it deals with risk factors for chronic diseases and injuries so that groups with the highest death rates receive larger benefits.

Additional Information

Please access these Web sites via the online version of this summary at http://dx.doi.org/10.1371/journal.pmed.0030260.

- A Perspective article by Gregory Pappas in this issue of PLoS Medicine (DOI: 10.1371/journal.pmed.0030357) discusses the methods of this piece of research and the findings
- The American Medical Students' Association deals with the question "What are Health Disparities?" on its web site
- The National Institutes of Health's "Strategic Research Plan to Reduce and Ultimately Eliminate Health Disparities" may be seen at the NIH web site
- The Office of Minority Health at the Centers for Disease Control and Prevention has a Web page called "Eliminating Racial and Ethnic Health Disparities"
- The issue of health inequalities in the US has also been dealt with by the Robert Wood Johnson Foundation

Appendix D

Community Approaches to Addressing Health Disparities

Carol Horowitz, M.D., M.P.H.[1]
Edward F. Lawlor, Ph.D.[2]

INTRODUCTION

A major national enterprise has grown up since the Institute of Medicine (IOM) report devoted to documenting health disparities; understanding their clinical, service, and social determinants; and mounting specific projects that address particular combinations of health status and racial and ethnic populations. This work has given extraordinary visibility to the existence of significant and stubborn disparities and mobilized an impressive number of university centers, provider groups, and community partners. Significant federal and private foundation funding has mapped onto this agenda. A great deal of innovation and adaptation has been spawned in this field, most notably the establishment and federal support for a broad body of community-based participatory research. Important state policy initiatives, such as the recently enacted Massachusetts Health Reform, have specific governance and accountability for disparities reductions.

Despite the number and variety of health disparities initiatives, there is growing restlessness that this enterprise is not yielding effective and scalable approaches and, most importantly, evidence of significant outcomes (Lurie and Fremont, 2006). For example, the Centers for Disease Control and Prevention's (CDC's) recent interim report on Healthy People 2010 worried that among the 195 disparities objectives there has only been

[1]Assistant Professor, Departments of Health Policy and Medicine, Mount Sinai School of Medicine.
[2]Dean and the William E. Gordon Professor, George Warren Brown School of Social Work, Washington University in St. Louis.

measurable improvements in 24 categories, declines in 14, and no change in 157 (CDC, 2007).

A number of concerns underlie this restlessness:

- Many initiatives do not embody the kind of community voice, support, and participation that is necessary for sustainable long-term results.
- Many initiatives are divorced from other significant community-development strategies that have the potential to influence the known determinants of health disparities (e.g., housing, safety, education, and civic engagement).
- Many initiatives are not built on a platform of governance, management, and adequate stable financing that assures a continuity of response from prevention, to early detection, to treatment, and to evaluation.

In simple terms, these initiatives have developed along two different paths. One broad approach to disparity reduction involves essential clinical services and interventions, generally developed by health status or diagnostic categories and supported by categorically clinical funding streams. Thus, a huge number of specific health disparities programs have emerged to address asthma, diabetes, breast and cervical cancers, cardiovascular disease, and other conditions. These programs have the advantage of being targeted to known disparities, can be tailored to provider and community resources, and have the potential to pursue evidence-based strategies. Often these programs are mounted by academic medical centers, health systems, or other provider organizations.

At the other end of the spectrum, an alternative set of community programs and policies proceed instead to address the socioeconomic "fundamentals" of community development and health. These initiatives, generally not on the radar of disparities researchers, are designed to enhance the strengths and assets that already exist in communities; to increase human, physical, and social capital; and to navigate complex processes of economic change (such as gentrification) in communities. These programs fall under the rubric of community building, community economic development, comprehensive community collaborations, and others in the so-called community-development field. Examples include the Local Initiative Support Corporation (LISC) and Community Builders.

For our purposes, however, many of these community-development approaches have significant health aspirations (sometimes explicit and sometimes implicit), often command huge investments and resources, as well as involve the same institutions—churches, schools, hospitals—and community leaders as community-based disparities programs. There is much to be learned about the overall impacts of these approaches, as well as their specific health consequences.

The thesis of this review for the IOM is that the "action" in community approaches to addressing health disparities lies in better understanding, design, and implementation of "hybrid" approaches to community development and health disparities. We define hybrid approaches as those derived from a combination of clinical, community, and other heterogeneous sources such as public health and policy. The best of these approaches have the virtue of empowering and mobilizing community resources and residents, but at the same time implementing systematic, sustainable, and clinically sound approaches to health behavior, screening, prevention and promotion, and treatment. Admittedly, the knowledge base for this assertion is thin; in fact, we believe one of the key frontiers in this field lies in creating an evidence-based approach, yielding results for community development that build off of the knowledge base about *both* community and health disparities that is more purposeful about evaluation and accomplishes better sharing and translation of information across disciplines and stakeholders.

DISPARITIES IN A COMMUNITY CONTEXT

Although many concepts and constructs of community abound, this paper treats communities as largely geographical or spatial units, though only as the best proxy for capturing a set of social relations and social institutions.[3] This means that we are largely concerned with so-called place-based approaches to health disparities and aligned with the literature on neighborhood or area effects on health (Diez Roux, 2001; Sampson, 2003).

A large literature focused on the role of socioeconomic and community factors in health outcomes has grown up in social science, public health, and the field of community organization and development. The backdrop to this literature on community effects is an even larger literature on the socioeconomic determinants of racial and ethnic health disparities. The pathways by which socioeconomic position and resources affect health status are well understood in concept, but more difficult to attribute empirically. Education, for example, provides opportunities for certain occupational pathways, which in turn produce different income streams, occupational exposure to health hazards, wherewithal to engage in positive health behaviors, and access to communities and social networks that are believed to reinforce health behaviors. Perceptions of racial discrimination, for example, have been linked across a large body of studies to

[3]For a complete discussion and review of different concepts of community see Robert Chaskin (1997).

health behavior, physical health, and mental health, although the precise mechanisms for how discrimination translates into physical or behavioral outcomes via stress or other pathways is less well established empirically (Williams et al., 2003).

The state of the evidence about these socioeconomic pathways to health disparities is crucial to the justification of community approaches. If policy and programs can in fact systematically affect social variables such as education, employment, or housing, and these improvements translate into health outcomes, then we have the beginnings of a model for influencing significant health disparities at the community level. However, the empirical understanding of how these socioeconomic mechanisms work at the community level is still quite limited. Nonetheless, many observers believe that research and policy experimentation specifically devoted to influencing these indirect socioeconomic pathways to health disparities should proceed apace. Alegría et al. (2003), for example, have argued that interventions in schooling, housing, and income support (earned income tax credits) are empirically defensible and justified in the field of mental health disparities. Adler and Newman's conclusion about the role of social capital in generating health outcomes is similar: "The literature on social capital has not yet explained why neighborhoods with similar demographics differ on social cohesion and trust, or established whether social capital is stable. But the associational evidence between social trust and health outcomes is striking and suggests that these are complementary frontiers worthy of exploration for addressing health issues along with raising income or educational attainment" (Adler and Newman, 2002, p. 67).

The literature on community effects on health disparities demonstrates that many community factors contribute to differential health outcomes by race and ethnicity, over and above individual characteristics (Bigby, 2007). A recent annotated bibliography of this literature by itself runs 93 pages long.[4] The sources of these community influences are numerous and complex, including risks created by the built environment such as lead in housing, access to the "ingredients" of healthy living such as affordable healthy foods, lack of community resources such as parks and green spaces that promote activity, ambient levels of stressors such as violence that may have physical and psychological sequlae, and disadvantages in access and in quality of health services and public health supports.

Despite the extent of this literature, again there is relatively little rigorous empirical evidence that demonstrates the mechanisms by which community characteristics or the ways in which community interventions produce observable differences in health outcomes. In part, this stems from

[4]For a review of this literature see Rebecca Flournoy and Irene Yen, *The Influence of Community Factors on Health* (PolicyLink, 2004).

the daunting statistical and data requirements for sorting out the multiple influences on health—the selection of individuals (with given health characteristics) into neighborhoods in the first place, the necessity for broad and multiple levels of data, and the substantial need for statistical variation across communities and groups, especially in nonexperimental data (Duncan and Raudenbush, 2001; Kawachi and Berkman, 2003).

The most intriguing recent empirical evidence of community-level effects *per se* comes from the Move to Opportunity (MTO) demonstration, in which 4,600 families in public housing in five cities were randomly assigned to different treatment groups of housing options and community environments. Adults in the experiment showed significant improvements in mental health and reductions in obesity with moves to new and higher-income communities; teenage girls showed improvements in mental health and reductions in risky behavior. Interestingly, teenage boys exhibited increases in risky behaviors relative to the control group (Kling and Liebman, 2004). Residents in individual MTO sites have shown substantial declines in specific health outcomes that need medical attention, such as injuries and asthma attacks. Other studies involving movers to new communities from distressed public housing, the so-called HOPE VI studies, however, have not yet shown improvements in health status, despite extraordinarily high rates of chronic and mental health conditions at baseline in this population. (Harris and Kaye, 2004; Manjarrez et al., 2007).

The critical role of community-level factors in addressing health disparities has led some commentators to argue that communities should become the "unit of analysis" for interventions, and community development should become the broad framework for implementing approaches (Robinson, 2005). Failure to make communities the unit of analysis means that a number of opportunities to design innovative and effective approaches are lost. First, most disparities of interest have important "nonhealth" community predispositions—environment, levels of community violence, and so on. Second, many disparities represent mixtures of social and health factors that cannot be easily disentangled into a simple clinical intervention. High rates of obesity and diabetes in communities reflect such a complex bundle of medical, health behavior, mental health, community resources, and access to health care. Third, many interventions require the active participation of community residents in order to be effective; this participation cannot be imposed. Fourth, many disadvantaged communities simultaneously exhibit health disparities because of the coexistence of poverty, racial concentration and segregation, and lack of access to health and other key supports. In the city of Chicago, for example, a relatively small number of disadvantaged neighborhoods on the south and west sides exhibit the highest rates of asthma, cancer, heart disease, sexually transmitted infections, diabetes, deaths from injuries and violence, and other critical health outcomes. Even in the face of this overlapping epidemiology, "siloed" approaches to health disparities miss the opportunity to marshal large-scale community participation and resources to design approaches that sweep at least across interrelated health-related conditions—for example, substance use, violence, high-risk sexual behavior—in a community.

A MULTILEVEL FRAMEWORK

As shown in Figure D-1, there have historically been two paths toward addressing the health needs of individuals in communities. In the clinical setting, interventions improve health care processes and outcomes, but there is limited evidence of their impact on health disparities. In the community setting, interventions improve community status, but there is limited evidence of their impact on health. Policy and public health interventions can influence health through clinical or community settings, and may address health directly.

Over the past decade, in recognition of the inadequate improvements in minority health, clinical, policy, public health, and community leaders have begun to consider what we will call a hybrid approach to health improvement, namely integrating features of clinical, community, and other (i.e., public health) approaches to address both biological and social determinants of health. These hybrid approaches can be focused in communities or in clinical settings, but the expertise of both is brought to bear on the problem, the solution, the evaluation, and plans for dissemination and sustainability. We compare their features in Table D-1. Following the table, we provide an overview of clinical and community approaches to disparities. We then discuss the issues and opportunities for advancing hybrid approaches. Finally, we conclude with a set of ideas about how hybrid approaches might be organized and implemented at scale.

CLINICALLY DRIVEN APPROACHES

Without question, the effective therapies developed and tested using basic science, clinical, and health services research have significantly contributed to improving the life expectancy of Americans of all racial and ethnic backgrounds. Yet, these diagnostic and therapeutic breakthroughs and unprecedented health care spending have not resulted in elimination of health care or health disparities for the majority of health conditions, even among populations with equal access to care. Several shortcomings of the current approach may help explain this disconnect. Table D-2 shows the building blocks of clinically oriented research to improve health. After each are descriptions of potential missteps that may occur if clinical interven-

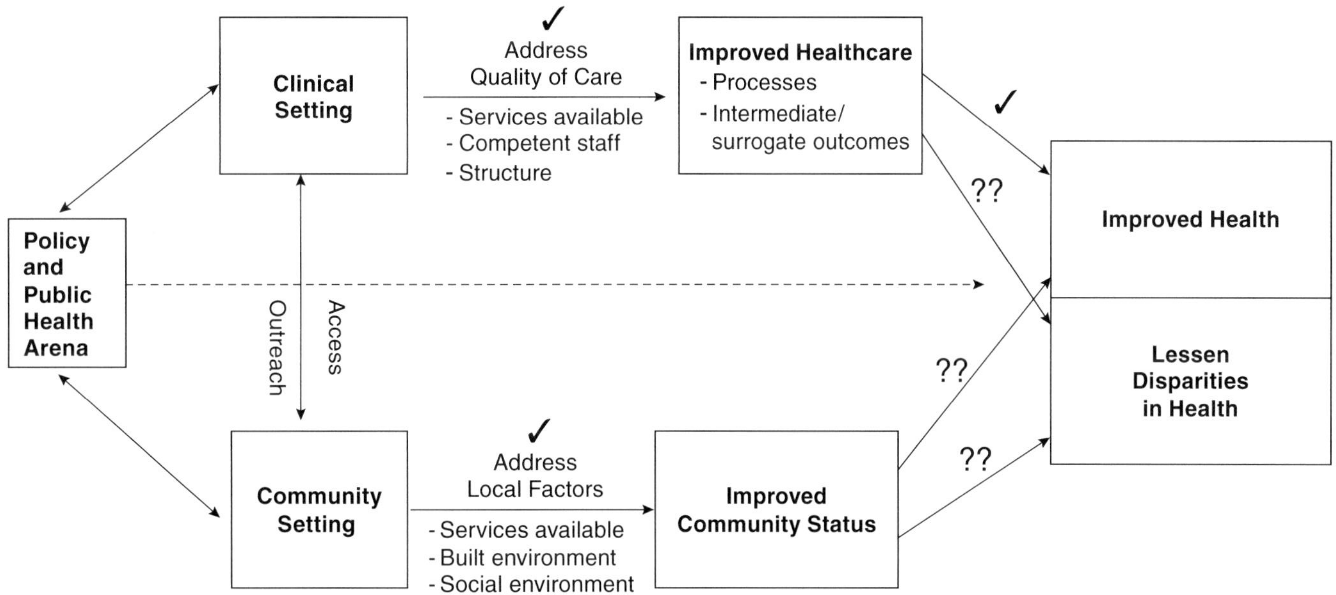

FIGURE D-1 Clinical and community approaches to health.

TABLE D-1 Characteristics of Clinical, Hybrid, and Community Interventions to Improve Health

Level	Clinical	Hybrid	Community
Intervention locus	Health care settings and related organizations	Centered clinically or in the community, but combine efforts from both disciplines	Neighborhoods, or nongeographically defined communities
Theory for health improvement	Evidence base of impact of clinical interventions on health	Simultaneously addressing clinical and community factors will have more direct and lasting impact	Improve community factors (social, economic, environmental, political) and health will also improve
Advantages	Address biological determinants of health; proven impact on health; enhance clinical resources and capacity	Address biological and social determinants of health; sustainable designs; enhance community and clinical resources and capacity	Address social determinants of health; sustainable designs; enhance community resources and capacity
Disadvantages	Limited evidence of impact on reducing disparities in health outcomes; employ narrow clinical perspective; challenges for sustainability and effectiveness (beyond efficacy)	Limited evidence of impact on health outcomes; interventions often local, may be challenging to scale up; time-consuming, intensive to initiate	Limited evidence of any health impact; target-efficiency problem (target broad, timeframe long, not specific for health)
Feasibility of implementation	Feasible in tightly controlled settings	Feasible with adequate development time and collaboration	Feasible with adequate infrastructure, resources and large-scale collaborations
Challenges of translation/replication	Translation to routine practice may be difficult	Replication may be difficult due to strong local influences	Both may be difficult given size and scope

TABLE D-2 Steps in Isolated Clinical Research Addressing Health Disparities and Their Pitfalls

Research Step	Pitfall If Lack Community Partnership	Potential Impact of Pitfall
Identify concerns	Look through narrow clinical lens. Patient/community ideas and priorities not taken into account. Do not look at social determinants of health.	Identified reasons for health disparities do not adequately explain disparities. Overlook novel areas for assessment and intervention.
Design study	Design lacks combination of cultural and evaluative competence. Target population may not be interested in participating, study may not be relevant.	Increased likelihood of negative study.
Identify sites, recruit patients	Inconvenient locations for patients. Sites chosen do not include epicenters of illness (site convenient, not relevant). Steps not taken to build trust. Recruitment strategies not motivational.	Poor recruitment/response rates. Fail to target the most appropriate population.
Assess processes	Labeled successes may not impact outcomes. Omit qualitative evaluations. Do not solicit evaluations by subjects.	Increased screening, contact with health care or surveillance, not clear if improved health. Unable to identify or act on study shortcomings.
Assess outcomes	Find no outcome improvement due to earlier flaws.	Missed opportunity. "Blame the victim": lack of improvement is patient's fault.
Disseminate impact	Disseminate scientifically but not to community. Community does not have ability to act on results. Results not used to inform/influence policy.	Reinforce "drive-by research" attitude held by community. Lost opportunity to capitalize on benefits beyond the specific project.
Sustain intervention	Interventions not designed with sustainability in mind.	Benefit disappears along with funding.

tions are conducted in isolation from the wider sociocultural context where patients spend the vast majority of their lives.

Two examples of the incomplete impact of clinical research merit further description: breast cancer treatment and diabetes prevention. Breast cancer is an area where disparities in processes, namely screening, often using community-centered education, appear to be narrowing, yet disparities in breast cancer deaths persist (Dietrich et al., 2006; Earp et al., 2002; Erwin et al., 1999; Smith-Bindman et al., 2006; Weir et al., 2003). Minority women with early-stage breast cancer are far less likely to receive necessary adjuvant treatments, even when equally referred to oncologists (Bickell et al., 2006). Perhaps the simpler process (mammography) is easier to address than is breast cancer treatment, which requires a multidisciplinary approach. Perhaps women of color also face disproportionate nonclinical barriers to treatment.

Diabetes is another area in which clinicians and clinical researchers are making strides and yet persons of color do not appear to reap sufficient benefits. Minority individuals are more likely to develop and die from diabetes, and disparities in death between whites and blacks/Latinos are widening (Mokdad et al., 2003). If prevention efforts are not developed and widely implemented, one in two black and Latino children born this decade will develop diabetes, as opposed to one in four whites (Narayan et al., 2003). Several clinically based programs, most notably the large, multisite Diabetes Prevention Program, found that weight loss among overweight adults with pre-diabetes can prevent or delay diabetes (Knowler et al., 2002). In this program, weight loss even eliminated racial and ethnic disparities in incident diabetes. Despite this unusually promising result, the program has been neither expanded, nor continued, even at the sites where its effectiveness was proven. Less expensive methods are needed to achieve the degree of weight loss and diabetes prevention seen in this costly, time-consuming efficacy trial (Eddy et al., 2005).

COMPREHENSIVE COMMUNITY-DEVELOPMENT APPROACHES

Community-development and community-building approaches emphasize the development of community capacity and community connections as the means to producing better outcomes such as economic opportunity, safety, housing conditions, and health status (Chaskin et al., 2001). Community-building approaches tend to emphasize local leadership development, promotion of collaborations, strengthening the capacity of community-based organizations, strengthening of social capital, and generation of new resources for housing and economic development.

A classic example of a comprehensive community-development approach based on a community-building philosophy would be initiatives supported by the LISC:

> LISC helps resident-led, community-based development organizations transform distressed communities and neighborhoods into healthy ones—good places to live, do business, work and raise families. By providing capital, technical expertise, training and information, LISC supports the development of local leadership and the creation of affordable housing, commercial, industrial and community facilities, businesses and jobs. (LISC, 2006)

These community-building programs individually and collectively represent substantial commitments of public and private resources, as well as community leadership and effort. LISC alone claims to have mobilized over $7.8 billion for projects in 300 urban and rural communities (LISC, 2006). Development banks, such as ShoreBank, or commercial banks with large community-development portfolios, represent significant sources of capital and expertise. Bank of America, for example, expects to invest $750 billion in community economic development over the next 10 years. Major foundations, such as Ford, McArthur, and Kellogg, have also built their strategy and funding priorities around these comprehensive community-development initiatives, in most cases leveraging an additional set of federal and state development resources. These sums dwarf the scale of most disparities interventions, yet there seems to be little effort devoted to capture and leverage these resources to strategically improve environment and community capacity in ways that produce measurable health outcomes.

On the whole, these comprehensive community-building initiatives and the national health disparities agendas have proceeded on largely separate tracks. While the connections of community-building initiatives and the efforts of public health and disparities programs operating in communities may seem self-evident, a recent review by Kieffer and Reischman (2004) concludes that the "reality is that many public health interventions are not coupled with community building strategies; and many groups undertaking community building do not include measures of improved public health as an outcome of their activities" (p. 2).

The implications of this disconnect are significant. Health disparities initiatives by themselves cannot command the level of resources and community attention necessary to impact the myriad of physical, social, and economic factors that underlie community health outcomes. Since community leadership and institutions are critical to the success of any health intervention, it may be necessary for community health interventions to become aligned with these larger community-development efforts to be able to capture the necessary time and attention.

There are a number of good reasons why community health approaches to disparities reduction have not been built on this platform of comprehensive community building. First, these approaches tend to emphasize the community process over interventions and implementation. In this world, collaborations, connections, relationship building, partnerships, and process often take precedence over specific interventions and implementation. Second, these approaches vest enormous control with community residents and stakeholders to define their own assets and approaches, whatever the views of experts may be. Particular health disparities may or may not rise to the top of the community hierarchy of priorities and needs for attention and resources. Third, by the very nature of comprehensive community approaches, these initiatives may have low target efficiency for a particular health condition. Efforts to improve employment, education, safety, and other community factors may have marginal or indirect effects on a particular health condition of interest. Finally, these comprehensive collaborations are often slow and halting in their progress and observable outcomes.

HYBRID APPROACHES (MIXED APPROACHES)

Hybrid approaches imply that community and clinical and other resources are both deployed and coordinated in developing and implementing programs to address health disparities. Interventions can be centered or grounded in one of five disciplines or areas: clinical, public health, policy, community, and research. We review existing approaches from these perspectives in the following sections.

Clinically Centered Hybrid Approaches

These approaches invite community, public health, policy, and research experts into the clinical setting in order to make clinical care more responsive to vulnerable populations (i.e., low-income individuals, or persons of color) and to make clinical interventions more effective in improving their health. Two approaches are gaining favor: systems redesign to make systems more culturally competent and effective, and health management and support to facilitate patient self-management and navigation.

Health Systems Redesign

Health systems leaders can look outside their clinical boundaries to find expertise and models to improve the care they deliver. Efforts are well under way to make health centers meet current standards for culturally and linguistically appropriate services (CLAS). Some translate materials into common languages and offer brief cultural sensitivity trainings. More comprehensive efforts also aim to include a well-trained and diverse staff and gain a deeper understanding of the populations they serve, and they use this understanding and active community input, creating a welcoming, educational, health-promoting clinical environment (Horowitz et al., 2000; National Standards for Culturally and Linguistically Appropriate Services in Health Care, 2001). Data on the impact of CLAS on health outcomes is scarce, although providing such basic services should not be considered controversial.

Broader approaches to providing health care in communities of color have been under way for decades. The community health center model that emerged as part of the war on poverty in fact targeted the roots of poverty by combining the resources of local communities with federal funds to establish neighborhood clinics. Because these centers are governed by community boards, and provide access regardless of ability to pay, there is some evidence that patients in these centers receive more timely screening and preventive services.

To combat the continued heavy burden of chronic illnesses at these centers, the Health Disparities Collaboratives of the Health Resources and Services Administration (HRSA) employed Wagner's Chronic Care Model, a system that encourages high-quality disease management (Landon et al., 2007; Wagner, 1998). The collaboratives significantly improved the processes of care for two of the three conditions studied (diabetes and asthma), but there was no improvement in the clinical outcomes studied. The authors reflect that "achieving improvements in both longer-term and intermediate outcomes may require more intensive interventions in order to overcome environmental factors that pose particular challenges for patients." As shown in Figure D-2, this model asserts that to improve the health of the population, health systems organizations reach out to form community alliances and partnerships with state programs, local agencies, schools, faith organizations, and businesses, a step those implementing the model may not have focused on adequately.

Health Management and Support

Health management and support reforms are often built around new professional and paraprofessional roles that connect with community residents. Examples include clinical disease managers, community health workers who are usually employed by health systems, and more independent peer educators. Each straddles the clinical and community realms with the goal of helping patients better manage their health.

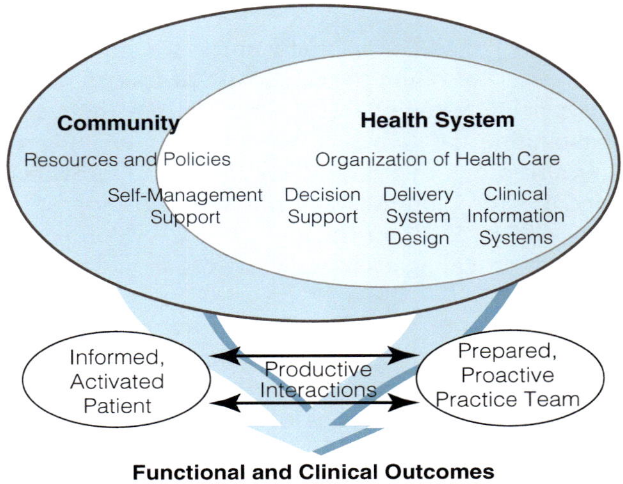

FIGURE D-2 Chronic care model.
SOURCE: Modified from Wagner (1998).

- *Disease managers* or nurse case managers work with patients who have specific, often chronic, health problems and they use information systems to track and monitor patients and clinical guidelines for care to improve both clinical and self-management (Norris et al., 2002). Initially developed to cut costs and resources, a new generation of these programs is culturally tailored to better educate, motivate, and support patients (Sisk et al., 2006). The programs have some strong effectiveness data in their favor, but current non-managed care payment structures that do not lead to cost savings for health systems if these relatively costly managers prevent hospitalizations may make it difficult to sustain these programs beyond the studies that prove their beneficial impact (Carryerou, 2006).
- *Community health workers* (CHWs) are lay community members who work with the local health care system, and usually share ethnicity, language, socioeconomic status, and life experiences with the community members they serve (HRSA, 2007). They can be members of the care delivery team (largely subordinate to a lead provider); navigators who assist individuals and families in negotiating complex service systems and bolster their clients' confidence when dealing with providers; screeners and health educators, often working with hard-to-reach populations; outreach workers, who reach individuals and families eligible for benefits or services and

persuade them to apply for help or come to a provider location for care; advocates for individual and community health needs; and organizers who become active in a community over a specific health issue, promoting self-directed change and community development. There are myriad evaluations of CHWs and the meta-analyses of these studies. CHW trials reveal significantly increased access to health care, improved asthma symptoms and decreased use of urgent care, blood pressure control, breast feeding, and decreased high-risk sexual behavior (Andrews et al., 2004; Brownstein et al., 2005; HRSA, 1998; Krieger et al., 2005; Lavery et al., 2005; Lewin et al., 2005; National Fund for Medical Education, 2006; Rosenthal, 1998). The CHW workforce is likely to increase in the forthcoming years (HRSA, 2007).

- *Peer educators* are distinguished from CHWs because they are more independent of the health care system. Lay-led, community-based peer-group sessions are an effective and cost-effective method to improve patients' self-management skills, health outcomes, and hospitalization rates. They use trained lay leaders with backgrounds and health problems similar to those of the participants, incorporating evidence of the effectiveness of role models in increasing patients' confidence in their ability to manage their conditions, and recognizing patient education should be inexpensive and widely available and that lay leaders from the community can impart information that may not be accepted from outsiders. These programs have significant health benefits in diabetes, asthma, seniors with heart disease, and with heterogeneous groups of persons with chronic conditions (Brown, 1999; Center for the Advancement of Health, 1996; Fries et al., 1998; Ladhenuso et al., 1996; Lorig and Gonzalez, 1992; Lorig et al., 1999, 2001; Mazzuca et al., 1986).

Policy-Centered/-Driven Hybrid Approaches

The two best examples of policy-driven hybrid approaches to community health disparities are the federal CDC Racial and Ethnic Approaches to Community Health (REACH) 2010 program and the California Healthy Communities Campaign.

REACH 2010

The CDC launched the REACH 2010 initiative in 1999 to address disparities in six priority areas: cardiovascular disease, immunizations, breast and cervical cancers screening, diabetes, HIV/AIDS, and infant mortality. Six racial and ethnic groups were designated for these programs: blacks,

American Indians, Alaskan Natives, Asian Americans, Hispanic Americans, and Pacific Islanders. By 2004, 40 separate projects were being supported under this initiative and evaluation results had begun to be disseminated.

Overall, the REACH 2010 projects emphasized local leadership and resident participation, prevention and education, and community-based participatory research. A variety of interventions and community approaches have been supported under the REACH framework. Bronx Health REACH, for example, involved 40 community-based organizations with a heavy emphasis on faith-based approaches to reducing rates of diabetes and related cardiovascular morbidity and mortality. In Oklahoma, the REACH project seeks to increase levels of physical activity with the ultimate goal of affecting diabetes and cardiovascular disease among tribal communities.

The theory of REACH's community participation and health outcomes is best depicted in their "logic model," which traces the connections between community awareness, coalition and community organization, community changes processes, health behavior changes, and health outcomes. In practice, REACH projects are expected to define the community coalitions and capacity, design, and intervention and tactics that have the basis to affect the targeted health outcome, produce community and community systems change, produce a significant amount of behavioral change, and ultimately reduce the observed disparity of interest.

Recently, data are beginning to appear on the effects of the REACH 2010 projects. Findings from the REACH Risk Factor Survey indicate significant gains in the proportion of blacks and Hispanics in REACH communities screened for cholesterol, the proportion of American Indians in REACH communities taking medications for high blood pressure, and the proportion of Asian American men in REACH communities who do not smoke (CDC, 2007).

For the purposes of this paper, the REACH projects represent a hybrid approach that attempts to take account of community coalitions and input, but with a systematic goal of reducing particular health disparities. In general, the REACH projects have involved a limited range of community participants and limited control over health provider and community-development resources. Most important, these approaches tend to tackle one condition at a time and, given resources and time, they eschew a larger approach to community development and change.

California Healthy Communities

At the state level, the most ambitious and integrative approach to health disparities reductions is the California Campaign to Eliminate Racial and Ethnic Disparities, and its affiliates the Prevention Institute and the Disparity Reducing Advances Project. The Campaign is directed at nine medical issues: cardiovascular disease, breast cancer, cervical cancer, diabetes, HIV/AIDS, infant mortality, asthma, mental health, and trauma. Philosophically, the campaign is dedicated to tackling fundamental causes of injury and illness. Its "logic model" envisions a progression to disparities that begins with root causes, behavioral and environmental factors, and access to quality health services. The Campaign seeks to be encompassing of a wide variety of actors, including public health, social services, education, cultural organizations, and community-based organizations.

The Campaign represents an impressive assembly of funding, collaborations, and knowledge resources. Funding has come from the California Endowment, the California Wellness Foundation, and Kaiser Permanente, as well as numerous other smaller grants and contracts. The principle leadership and collaboration has come from the American Public Health Association, the Prevention Institute, and the California Health and Human Services Agency. Leaders of the California Campaign liken it to some of the biggest and most visible campaigns of the modern era—the Marshall Plan and the Manhattan Project—as examples of the scale and unity of purpose that will be necessary to produce meaningful change in California's health status. Recently, leadership of the Campaign has paid considerable attention to social movements as a framework for mobilizing the political will and social change necessary to achieve the desired large-scale outcomes.

The California Campaign reflects many of the ingredients for a scalable disparities approach, significant funding, a powerful strategic focus, widespread collaboration, and a commitment to applying the knowledge base about effective interventions and community process. However, as even the leaders of this Campaign acknowledge, there is still a long way to go to produce a cohesive approach that capitalizes on other disparities experiences and involves the other sectors—such as urban and community planning, housing, and so forth—that have significant roles in addressing disparities at the community level. It remains to be seen how well this kind of highly orchestrated and systematic approach to disparities reduction will fare in giving communities voice and engaging the community in meaningful change processes to produce the kinds of large-scale statistical results that are envisioned in the campaign.

Research-Centered Hybrid Approaches in the Community

Researchers are now quite comfortable using secondary data analyses to study health disparities. It would be interesting for them to partner with community development, environmental development, and urban planning leaders, to conduct community-targeted secondary analyses, merging clinical and community-level data to study impacts of development on heath. These partnerships may help build the mutual understanding, trust, and respect needed among the various stakeholders to work on prospective projects to improve health.

Beyond the relative absence of evaluation findings from the wide range of existing disparities interventions, even less work has been done to estimate the economic value of these initiatives, either as a guide for resource allocation or for policy advocacy. A model of this work is the recent cost-effectiveness analysis of improved quality of diabetes care in Federally Qualified Neighborhood Health Care Centers (Huang et al., 2007). This analysis suggests that systematic improvements in diabetes care would be cost-effective for society because the overall health effects (lifetime incidence of blindness, kidney disease, and heart disease) offset the costs of health services improvements.

This form of economic analysis is just the beginning of a necessary agenda to value community-based interventions to reduce disparities. In many respects, cost-benefit or cost-effectiveness analysis of this form of clinical service is the easiest case; broader-based or hybrid approaches will require much more effort and sophistication to capture the full range of social costs and benefits. Indeed, many of the effects represent externalities in the economic sense and will not be typically priced or valued in traditional economic markets. Reducing the incidence of high lead levels, for example, yields a host of developmental, educational, and community benefits than extend beyond the simple accounting of health care costs and benefits. In traditional cost-benefit analysis, these outcomes typically fall in the domain of externalities and are not priced or valued in direct market exchanges, but they may represent the paramount economic benefit of community-level investments.

Being able to account for the return on investment of health disparities interventions is more akin to the literature and practice of social return on investment, where effects on the environment and the social opportunities of beneficiaries are central concerns (Olsen, 2003). Especially in cases where disparities approaches have the character of hybrid clinical and community-development initiatives, considerable attention will need to be paid to developing methodology, collecting data, and reporting results in forms that are appropriate to the task.

Creating a New Cadre of Community-Based Researchers

In this young field, there is only emerging evidence of the health benefits accrued with a community focus. Little is known about the relative effectiveness of different organizational strategies to build the enterprises needed for this work. Building a cadre of professional and lay experts to conduct and evaluate interventions will take time, yet there is tremendous opportunity for leadership development, such as the new emphasis in the Robert Wood Johnson Clinical Scholars Program.

Critical to the advance and credibility of this field will be the involvement of new investigators and an expansion of the pool of community-based researchers. Venues to train new community and academically based investigators in community-based participatory research (CBPR) are expanding. There are also many reviews, guides, and literature syntheses available to guide individuals through the steps to conducting CBPR.[5] To build new opportunities and expertise in the field, areas to consider include the following:

- Creating formal liaison centers to allow community representatives to better understand research, better define their concerns and find researchers they can work with, and for researchers to learn about CBPR and link with community representatives
- Creation of clearer mechanisms for academic advancement to legitimize CBPR and to ensure that talented researchers are supported to remain in the field (Commission on Community-Engaged Scholarship in the Health Professions, 2005)
- Institutional sponsorship of community–academic partnerships at the highest level
- Identification of mentors for community and academic partners locally and nationally (Community Campus Partnerships on Health maintains a database of community partners for this purpose)
- Creation of an information clearinghouse on disparities that networks individuals, programs, and opportunities, houses databases with information on local and regional health and health disparities and relevant community characteristics, and lists community-based disparities reduction programs and links to their evaluations
- Finding new mechanisms to increase interaction among social scientists, medical investigators, public health, and community-development scholars in the pursuit of a community-level knowledge base leading to effective interventions

Taking Advantage of Large-Scale Translational Research Opportunities (Bench to Bedside to Barrio)

Historically, translational research has focused on "bench to bedside" (Zerhouni, 2003). Acknowledging the slow trajectory toward eliminating health disparities and the failure of those few programs that show promise to be sustained or disseminated, a new term has emerged in translational

[5]See http://depts.washington.edu/ccph/index.html.

research circles: "bench to bedside to barrio." Regional and national efforts have started bringing together federal and private funders with academic and community leaders to identify barriers to and enablers of effective community–academic research partnerships and to develop and disseminate guidelines and best practices for conducting community-based clinical and translational research in minority communities. They help coordinate support for developing and maintaining core research infrastructure to enable community participation, developing research protocols that work effectively in community settings, and building community buy-in and trust to enhance recruitment and retention of research participants.[6]

The best funded and most visible of such programs are the new Clinical and Translational Science Awards (CTSAs), a new consortium to transform how clinical and translational research is conducted, ultimately enabling researchers to provide new treatments more efficiently and quickly to patients. The consortium will link about 60 institutions to encourage development of new research methods, tools, and approaches; improve training and mentoring; assemble interdisciplinary research teams; and forge new partnerships with private and public health care organizations. According to the CTSA literature,[7] "CTSAs represent a new culture of translational healthcare research in which community engagement is key to success." The CTSA Community Engagement Steering Committee (one of eight subcommittees to coordinate institution topic-specific efforts with the national CTSA consortium) is charged with ensuring the successful implementation of a broad community-engagement plan among the CTSA sites by sharing knowledge, expertise, and resources and by effectively engaging communities in the translational research process via bidirectional dialogues. Their aims are (1) to find ways to get bench scientists and clinicians interested in priorities identified by communities; (2) to identify effective strategies to convince academic institutions that community engagement is important and deserves a supportive atmosphere (including adequate budgetary resources and influencing the National Institutes of Health culture to value community engagement and CBPR, collaborative budgeting strategies); and (3) to develop milestones for community engagement and research, including establishing boards, leveraging partnerships for funding, developing a registry of community-generated research ideas and needs, and developing outcomes and metrics for this research.

Taking Advantage of Public Health

Ever since the IOM report, *The Future of Public Health*, public health professionals and organizations have been looking to lead and participate

[6]See http://www.ncrr.nih.gov/research_infrastructure.
[7]See http://www.ctsaweb.org/commengage.html.

in disparities initiatives in a meaningful way. The IOM report defined a mission for public health of "assuring conditions in which people can be healthy," with its "aim to generate organized community effort . . . by applying scientific and technical knowledge to prevent disease and promote health" (IOM, 1988). The Committee recommended a host of activities that would position public health agencies and professionals in the middle of policy development, data collection and research, and capacity building to affect health status. Included in this agenda were issues of indigent health care, mental health, and environmental health. Schools of public health figured prominently in this agenda, and they were expected to cross boundaries with medicine, the social sciences, and other disciplines with the ultimate goal of generating new and effective interventions. Public health was envisioned to play a strong policy role with extensive interaction with government, social service agencies, and "street-level" contacts.

Without question, considerable progress has been made in the past 20 years in realizing this vision for public health, and many examples exist of the kind of collaborative, integrated approach that was envisioned by the IOM process. The CDC's STEPS program, directed at high-priority disparities issues of obesity, diabetes, and asthma, for example, embodies most of the principles of this IOM report. It seeks to implement an integrated approach at the community level that involves schools, employers, and other stakeholders; it attempts to affect policy and fundamental health behaviors; and it incorporates a strong evaluative component. However, in the scheme of disparities challenges, STEPS is a relatively modest public health initiative, allocating $44 million in fiscal year 2005 for 40 community projects.

While the agenda articulated in 1988 would seem to place public health departments, schools, and professionals at the heart of the disparities, few observers would conclude that public health has played the kind of overall leadership, integrative function, and applied community role that is necessary to effectuate significant changes in health disparities. Much has happened during this period, including funding challenges, the demand for homeland security and bioterrorism roles for public health, and other claims on public health's mission and priorities. Many movements are afoot to bring public health into a more central role, including a great deal of discussion about the role of public health in influencing the built environment in health disparities. The California Campaign represents an initiative that embodies both the philosophical commitment to prevention of a public health perspective as well as the professional and organizational leadership of the American Public Health Association. The research opportunities provided in CTSAs, Disparities Centers, and other large-scale initiatives may be important factors in bringing at least academic public health into a stronger and more applied community role in reducing health disparities.

Solving Organization, Finance, and Policy for Hybrid Approaches

Efforts to mount a systematic approach to racial and ethnic disparities at the community level are hampered by governance, funding, and management challenges of the health delivery system utilized by racial and ethnic minorities.

Governance

Especially since the demise of health planning in the 1980s, most areas of the country have no accountable party and no organized mechanism for governing health resources across the spectrum of public health, hospital systems, community health centers, and the myriad of private health providers and resources that are necessary for building effective health disparities collaborations. Governance of health is fragmented into different levels of administration (e.g., city, county, state), "fiefdoms" of health provision (e.g., public health versus hospitals), as well as different geographic jurisdictions. St. Louis, for example, is an agglomeration of 97 municipalities and a complex web of city, county, and state (both Illinois and Missouri) jurisdictions.[8] It is hard to overestimate the significance of these kinds of political, administrative, and even statistical fragmentations for mounting strategic approaches to disparities. This lack of overarching governance means that the most basic elements of a strategic approach—collecting data, creating a continuity of screening, prevention, and care—are dauntingly difficult administratively.

Funding

Health care interventions to address disparities are financed through a bewildering array of public and private resources. Some of these resources flow from categorical grants and contracts specifically targeted to fund a program or agency dedicated to a particular health outcome such as infant mortality. HRSA funding of specific Health Start programs, such as programs to improve the systems of care for pregnant women experiencing domestic or family violence, would be an example of a highly targeted discrete funding stream. Some of the financing flows to public and private providers such as payments (grants or fee for service) to Federally Qualified Health Centers or other community-based clinics. Some of the relevant resources flow through either traditional Medicaid or Medicaid waiver schemes. Some of the resources flow through county or city public hospital and clinic systems. Some services and costs are simply unfunded,

---

[8]See, for example, Terry Jones, *Fragmented by Design* (Jones, 2000).

meaning that cross-subsidies from charity care, disproportionate share, or philanthropic sources need to be found. An example of the consequences of this patchwork of financing can be seen in programs to reduce racial and ethnic disparities in breast cancer: projects have been successful in motivating women to be screened but have often struggled to find and pay for mammography services, as well as timely follow-up care. This follows directly from the fragmentation of financing and services. The providers and payment for community health promotion are often disconnected from the providers and payment for mammography and advanced cancer care.

Many disparities interventions are funded through research mechanisms whose short timeframes (usually 2–5 years) often preclude the development of substantive partnerships and do not allow for sustaining partnerships or successful interventions. This stuttering funding can only lead to transient improvements in health for small populations and mounting distrust of community members who view such endeavors as academic fodder.

In order to create the combination of resources, as well as continuity of service for community residents, much greater attention will need to be paid to the governance and financing of disparities approaches. At a minimum, this means that some form of regional data collection, coordination, and accountability for disparities interventions much be accomplished. It also means that payers and providers will need to be vested in the financing and outcomes of disparities initiatives. The Massachusetts health reform provides this kind of recognition of the integral role of financing and governance, but it too has been criticized for not backing up the rhetoric of a disparities priority with hard sources of funding.

Critical to commanding the resources and instruments to address the environmental, housing, educational, employment, and social service correlates of health disparities will be a recognition that larger-scale public policy is a key element of the disparities agenda. The best spokesperson for this perspective has been Margaret Alegría, who has argued that much of the action in hybrid approaches lies in understanding and policy reform of such programs as the Earned Income Tax Credit and Special Education (Alegría et al., 2003). Key policy areas that will affect the course of disparities approaches include public housing transformation, changes in the Community Reinvestment Act Provisions, welfare reform, immigration policy, Medicaid, and health care coverage. Typically, advocates and investigators do not see such large-scale social policy issues as part of the set of disparities levers and concerns, but the resources involved and implications for communities dominate many of the research-driven projects that have come to define the disparities field.

MODELS AND IDEAS FOR HYBRID COMMUNITY APPROACHES

In order to bring these hybrid approaches to scale, new community infrastructure and resources will need to be developed. Current approaches are typically small in scale, do not leverage significant resources, and do not capitalize on information and technical expertise. Creating scalable community approaches will require solutions to the financing problems inherent in many disparities initiatives. Community approaches that can be evaluated and that demonstrate statistical impact on disparities will also need to account for much larger populations and bring much greater analytic sophistication than most current community examples. Five models or heuristics are presented to give examples of how new hybrid approaches might be configured in ways that address many of the shortcomings identified in this paper.

1. *Regional Health Authorities:* A number of regional authorities already exist at different levels of aggregation. The Westside Health Authority in Chicago, for example, has led a number of community-development and health disparities initiatives with full community participation and advocacy. The Regional Health Commission in St. Louis addresses a range of data, provider, and policy functions from the perspective of the region as a whole. Regional Health Authorities effectively configured for addressing disparities would need to capture a financing stream (most likely though a Medicaid assessment or all-payer program), and adopt a dedicated focus on disparities reductions for particular communities to be effective.
2. *Community Development Banks/Corporations:* While improvement of community health is one of the stated initiatives of many comprehensive community-development initiatives, in practice the goals and resources are more tightly defined by housing and economic-development measures. However, these institutions and investments represent large flows of capital and often intensive community involvement. Bank of America, for example, will invest $750 billion in the next 10 years in community development. Many of these investments occur in exactly the same communities with a high prevalence of health disparities conditions. To organize this combined health/community-development approach, new partnerships would need to be struck with institutions such as Shorebank, LISC, Bank of America, the Department of Housing and Urban Development (HUD); as well as other regional investors and developers. Many of these initiatives are organized around community-development corporations that provide an initial infrastructure and governance of these collaborations.

3. *University–Community Partnerships:* A number of successful university–community partnerships have been built in recent years, some with the formal support of HUD and other federal agencies. The major examples, the University of Pennsylvania and the University of Chicago, have largely focused on community economic development and urban schools. While there certainly are examples of academic medical centers and schools of public health that have significant community partnerships, they have not been organized and disciplined by a systematic approach to addressing disparities in particular communities. The emergence of CPBR, the emphasis on CTSAs, the community interest of academic public health, and the community training needs of many medical school make this an opportune time to consider scaling up and organizing university–community partnerships specifically for addressing disparities. To the extent that these partnerships can leverage the health care delivery system at major academic centers, there is also the potential to create more seamless structures of financing and health care service in these neighborhoods. These urban community models have the potential for not only addressing urban disparities but also utilizing university networks in rural health.
4. *CBPR Practice Networks:* As this appendix describes, one of the exciting developments in addressing disparities has been the number of projects and community relationships stimulated by CBPR. Despite the apparent early successes of this movement, it is operating at small scales and with little opportunity for cross-fertilization, data development, and comparative analysis. A structure that organizes and supports this movement across community sites has the potential to create a multiplier from these projects. A potential model for collaboration, data collection, and technical assistance are the national practice networks that are emerging in other areas of health services research. The extension of this idea to communities would involve the creation of comprehensive practice network structures and data and information systems at the community level. Even better, a consortium of community-based practice networks would allow better systematic and comparative evaluation of community-based disparities initiatives.
5. *Provider Networks or Systems to Address Disparities:* Many of the current priority conditions have a heavy reliance on improvements in access and quality of health services in low-income and minority neighborhoods. As a practical matter, sufficient funding and sufficient "market penetration" to create a statistical impact will require multiple health care plans, systems, and providers operating in consort. Versions of these arrangements have been created in

cities to address ambulatory care provision, indigent care, and special service needs such as trauma care. These networks of systems typically require dedicated payment streams and some governance from the local health departments, state public health, or other public agent. Payment streams have included Medicaid provider assessment schemes, use of Disproportionate Share dollars, or allocations of city, county, or state revenues. A model for organizing these networks to address place-based disparities would be the creation of special health disparities districts, analogous to medical districts, that would provide incentives for health plans to create new community-based programs as well as access and quality improvement in relevant services.

SUMMARY AND RECOMMENDATIONS

The central problem for building community approaches to reducing health disparities is to knit together community, provider, funding, and academic resources at such a scale that there is the potential to have statistical effects on population health outcomes. Many of the initiatives to date have demonstrated good will, effective community collaborations, and reasoned approaches to addressing disparities, but they tend to be fragmented, small in scale, and inadequately or transiently funded. Considering realistically the magnitude of behavioral change and service provision that is necessary to have a statistical impact on disparities, at the community level much less nationally, it will require a level of commitment and organization that far outstrips current models of intervention. In effect, the disparities initiatives need to be upsized from a cottage industry to substantial organization and scale.

Hybrid approaches to improving health outcomes and reducing disparities have the advantage of being clinically centered in the community, but they leverage the community participation, resources, and environmental agenda that are associated with broader community-development strategies. In principle these hybrid approaches have greater potential for sustainability and scale. They have the disadvantage of being diffuse, community process oriented, and difficult to target narrowly on specific disparities interventions. Many varieties of these hybrid approaches exist, such as the REACH 2010 and CBPR projects, but little empirical evidence about outcomes and little analysis of strategies are available for making these approaches successful, scalable, and sustainable.

Our analysis of current hybrid community approaches has identified a number of issues that need to be addressed to advance these clinical and community models. The goal of these hybrid models should be that they are simultaneously clinically excellent as well as community-responsive initiatives. Significant adaptation will need to occur in the clinical enterprise in order to have mutuality and successful collaboration in the community. Innovation in the forms and utilization of data will be necessary. New commitments to community-level evaluation, including some version of social return on investment, will be necessary to learn from and advocate for these community-level initiatives. A new cadre of appropriately trained community-based researchers, with expertise in the community disciplines and experience with the cultural, social, and political realities of working in communities will need to be trained. CTSA opportunities will need to be seized, so that that the community side of this roadmap is highly responsive to community values and interests, not merely an appendage to the traditional clinical research enterprise. The resources of public health—both governmental and academic—will need to be reassessed and more effectively deployed to advance this agenda of hybrid approaches. Finally, solutions to the organizational and financing gaps in disparities programs will need to be fashioned.

There are currently a large number of alternative community disciplines, professionals, and organizations laying claim to the community-development and disparities agenda. Community health, community building, community organization and planning, urban planning, public health, environmental health, social work, and others all see themselves as primary professional leaders in this movement. From the perspective of communities, academic centers, health providers, social service organizations, public health agencies, faith-based organizations, and a host of advocacy organizations are all seeking to partner and mount their own versions of disparities programming. Meanwhile, some of the largest players in community development, the banks and developers, are often outside of the discussion, financing, and implementation of disparities programs.

Community collaborations (e.g., CBPRs) show great promise in the struggle to eliminate disparities. They can identify root causes of disparities, build on local assets, devise novel, clinically, and environmentally sensible designs with sustainability in mind, inspire robust research participation, and disseminate results so they inform policy and inspire further introspection and change. They are also community-organizing and -development initiatives in their own right. However, models for partnership in the literature describe years of planning—building relationships and crafting fair rules of engagement before research and interventions begin in earnest. While these processes must not be overlooked and local adaptation may be necessary for many interventions, the CBPR community must challenge itself to move from community-based planning (CBP) to "CBPR" with more efficiency and to find models that are proven to improve health and that can be exported to other communities or within the community, to address other health-related issues.

The solution is not to choose one or another of these community players as primary. Rather, new mechanisms which bring together some of these stakeholders in partnership with community residents and with focus on substantial disparities programming will be necessary. Examples we have considered include regional health authorities, community-development corporations, university–community partnerships, CBPR practice networks, and new forms of health plan districts or networks.

Our analysis has produced a beginning agenda for the IOM Roundtable to pursue in building better linkages between community development and clinical services—hybrid approaches—in the name of reducing disparities.

- Convene community-development organizations and funders, along with health disparities academic and practice leadership to design hybrid approaches.
- Promote the creation of an evidence-based clearinghouse for information and technical assistance in community development for reduction in health disparities (such a clearinghouse could be mounted under the auspices of public, association, university or foundation organizations).
- Convene the major health systems to address staffing, programming, disease management, and community partnerships approaches to disparities.
- Influence the major existing clinical/research mechanisms—CBPR, CTSAs, REACH 2010—to leverage the full spectrum of community resources beyond the traditional scope of the clinical and research requirements of these mechanisms.
- Commission a set of briefing papers that describe replicable models of community finance (e.g., disproportionate share hospital payment approaches), governance (e.g., health authorities), and communications innovations for effective and sustainable disparities reduction in communities.
- Reexamine the framework and recommendations of the IOM report *The Future of Public Health* with the goal of reinvigorating a public health agenda in community and health disparities.
- Convince a leading public health, health services, or community-development journal to publish a special issue on *methods* for evaluating community interventions and initiatives to reduce disparities—geographical and Health Impact Analysis, cost benefit and social return on investment analysis, multilevel and social network methods—as well as qualitative approaches.
- Engage a leading foundation in supporting the training and professional development of a new cadre of community-savvy academic leaders in the field of health disparities.

- Identify and encourage a set of universities with the academic mission, resources, and community context to seriously and systematically build hybrid approaches that bring the same sophistication to community engagement and partnership that they brought to other dimensions of translational science.

REFERENCES

Adler, N. E., and K. Newman. 2002. Socioeconomic disparities in health: Pathways and policies. *Health Affairs* 21(2):60–76.

Alegría, M., D. J. Pérez, and S. Williams. 2003. The role of public policies in reducing mental health status disparities for people of color. *Health Affairs* 22:51–64.

Andrews, J. O., G. Felton, M. E. Wewers, and J. Heath. 2004. Use of community health workers in research with ethnic minority women. *Journal of Nursing Scholarship* 36(4):358–365.

Bickell, N. A., J. J. Wang, S. Oluwole, D. Schrag, H. Godfrey, K. Hiotis, J. Mendez, and A. A. Guth. 2006. Missed opportunities: Racial disparities in adjuvant breast cancer treatment. *Journal of Clinical Oncology* 24:1357–1362.

Bigby, J. A. 2007. The role of communities in eliminating health disparities. In *Eliminating healthcare disparities in America: Beyond the IOM report*, edited by R. A. Williams. Totowa, NJ: Humana Press.

Brown, S. A. 1999. Interventions to promote diabetes self-management: State of science. *Diabetes Education* 25(6 Suppl):52–61.

Brownstein, J. N., L. R. Bone, C. R. Dennison, M. N. Hill, M. T. Kim, and D. M. Levine. 2005. Community health workers as interventionists in the prevention of heart disease and stroke. *American Journal of Preventive Medicine* 29(5 Suppl 1):128–133.

Carreyrou, J. 2006. How a hospital stumbled across an Rx for Medicaid. *Wall Street Journal*, June 22.

CDC (Centers for Disease Control and Prevention). 2007. *Racial and ethnic approaches to community health (REACH) U.S.: Finding solutions to health disparities*. Atlanta, GA: CDC.

Center for the Advancement of Health (The Center for Health Studies of Group Health Cooperative of Puget Sound). 1996. *An indexed bibliography on self-management for people with chronic disease*. 1st ed. Washington, DC: Center for the Advancement of Health.

Chaskin, R. J. 1997. Perspectives on neighborhoods and community: A review of the literature. *Social Service Review* 7:521–547.

Chaskin, R. J., P. Brown, S. Venkatesh, and A. Vidal. 2001. *Building community capacity: Modern applications of social work*. New York: Aldine de Gruyter.

Commission on Community-Engaged Scholarship in the Health Professions. 2005. *Linking scholarship and communities. Report of the Commission on Community-Engaged Scholarship in the Health Professions*. Community Campus Partnerships for Health. http://depts.washington.edu/ccph/pdf_files/Commission%20Report%20FINAL.pdf (accessed April 10, 2007).

Dietrich, A. J., J. N. Tobin, A. Cassells, C. M. Robinson, M. A. Greene, C. H. Sox, M. L. Beach, K. N. DuHamel, and R. G. Younge. 2006. Telephone care management to improve cancer screening among low-income women. A randomized, controlled trial. *Annals of Internal Medicine* 144(8):563–571.

Diez Roux, A. V. 2001. Investigating neighborhood and area effects on health. *American Journal of Public Health* 91:1783–1789.

Duncan, G. J., and S. W. Raudenbush. 2001. Getting context right in quantitative studies of child development. In *The well-being of children and families*, edited by A. Thornton. Ann Arbor, MI: University of Michigan Press, pp. 356–383.

Earp, J. A., E. Eng, M. S. O'Malley. 2002. Increasing use of mammography among older, rural African American women: Results from a community trial. *American Journal of Public Health* 92:646–654.

Eddy, D. M., L. Schlessinger, and R. Kahn. 2005. Clinical outcomes and cost-effectiveness of strategies for managing people at high risk for diabetes. *Annals of Internal Medicine* 143:251–264.

Erwin, D. O., T. S. Spatz, R. C. Stotts, and J. A. Hollenberg. 1999. Increasing mammography practice by African Mareican women. *Cancer Practice* 7:78–85.

Fries, J. F., C. E. Koop, J. Sokolov, C. E. Beadle, and D. Wright. 1998. Beyond health promotion: Reducing need and demand for medical care. *Health Affairs* 17(2):70–84.

Harris, L. E., and D. R. Kaye. 2004. How are HOPE VI families faring? Health. A roof over their heads. *The Urban Institute* 5:1–7.

Horowitz, C. R., M. H. Davis, A. S. Palermo, and B. C. Vladeck. 2000. Approaches to eliminating sociocultural disparities in health. *Health Care Financing Review* 21:57–74.

HRSA (Health Resources and Services Administration). 1998. *Impact of community health workers on access, use of services, and patient knowledge and behavior*. Bureau of Primary Health Care, Health Resources and Services Administration, U.S. Department of Health and Human Services.

HRSA. 2007 (March). *The Community Health Worker National Workforce Study*. Bureau of Health Professions, Health Resources and Services Administration, U.S. Department of Health and Human Services.

Huang, E. S., Q. Zhang, S. E. S. Brown, M. L. Drum, D. O. Meltzer, and M. H. Chin. 2007. The cost-effectiveness of improving diabetes care in U.S. federally qualified community health centers. *Health Services Research* 42(6 Pt 1):2174–2193.

IOM (Institute of Medicine). 1988. *The future of public health*. Washington, DC: National Academy Press.

Jones, T. 2000. *Fragmented by design: Why St. Loius has so many governments*. St. Louis, MO: Palmerston and Reed Publishing Company.

Kawachi, I., and L. F. Berkman. 2003. *Neighborhoods and health*. New York: Oxford University Press.

Kieffer, E. C., and J. Reischmann. 2004. *Contributions of community building to achieving improved public health outcomes*. Washington, DC: The Aspen Institute.

Kling, J., and J. B. Liebman. 2004. *Experimental analysis of neighborhood effects on youth*. Working Papers, Princeton University, Woodrow Wilson School of Public and International Affairs, Center for Health and Wellbeing.

Knowler, W. C., E. Barrett-Connor, S. E. Fowler, R. F. Hamman, J. M. Lachin, E. A. Walker, D. M. Nathan, and Diabetes Prevention Program Research Group. 2002. Reduction in the incidence of type 2 diabetes with lifestyle intervention or metformin. *New England Journal of Medicine* 346(6):393–403.

Krieger, J. W., T. K. Takaro, L. Song, and M. Weaver. 2005. The Seattle-King County Healthy Homes Project: A randomized, controlled trial of a community health worker intervention to decrease exposure to indoor asthma triggers. *American Journal of Public Health* 95:652–659.

Ladhenuso, A. T., T. Haahtela, J. Herrala, T. Kava, K. Kiviranta, P. Kuusisto, E. Perämäki, T. Poussa, S. Saarelainen, and T. Svahn. 1996. Randomized comparison of guided self-management and traditional treatment of asthma over one year. *British Medical Journal* 312(7003):748–752.

Landon, B. E., L. S. Hicks, A. J. O'Malley, T. A. Lieu, T. Keegan, B. J. McNeil, and E. Guadagnoli. 2007. Improving the management of chronic disease at community health centers. *New England Journal of Medicine* 356(9):921–934.

Lavery, S. H., M. L. Smith, A. A. Esparaza, A. Hrushow, M. Moore, and D. F. Reed. 2005. The community action model: A community-driven model designed to address disparities in heath. *American Journal of Public Health* 95(4):611–616.

Lewin, S. A., J. Dick, P. Pond, M. Zwarenstein, G. Aja, B. van Wyk, X. Bosch-Capblanch, and M. Patrick. 2005. Lay health workers in primary care and community health. *Cochrane Database of Systematic Reviews*, Issue 1. Art. No.: CD004015. DOI: 10.1002/14651858. CD004015.pub2.

LISC (Local Initiatives Support Corporation). 2006. *Annual report*. http://www.lisc.org/docs/brochures/media/lisc_ar_2006.pdf (accessed April 10, 2007).

Lorig, K., and V. Gonzalez. 1992. The integration of theory with practice: A 12-year case study. *Health Education Quarterly* 19:355–368.

Lorig, K. R., D. S. Sobel, A. L. Stewart, B. W. Brown Jr., A. Bandura, R. Ritter, V. M. Gonzalez, D. D. Laurent, and H. R. Holman. 1999. Evidence suggesting that a chronic disease self-management program can improve health status while reducing hospitalization: A randomized trial. *Medical Care* 37:5–14.

Lorig, K. R., P. Ritter, A. L. Stewart, D. S. Sobel, B. W. Brown Jr., A. Bandura, V. M. Gonzalez, D. D. Laurent, and H. R. Holman. 2001. Chronic disease self-management program: 2-year health status and health care utilization outcomes. *Medical Care* 39:1217–1223.

Lurie, N., and A. Fremont. 2006. Looking forward: Cross-cutting issues in the collection and use of racial/ethnic data. *Health Services Research* 41:1519–1533.

Manjarrez, C. A., S. J. Popkin, and E. Guernsey. 2007. Poor health: Adding insult to injury for HOPE VI families. HOPE VI: Where do we go from here? *The Urban Institute* 5:1–9.

Mazzuca, S. A., N. H. Moorman, M. L. Wheeler, J.A. Norton, N. S. Fineberg, F. Vinicor, S. J. Cohen, and C. M. Clark Jr. 1986. The diabetes education study: A controlled trial of the effects of diabetes patient education. *Diabetes Care* 9(1):1–10.

Mokdad, A. H., E. S. Ford, B. A. Bowman, W. H. Dietz, F. Vinicor, V. S. Bales, and J. S. Marks. 2003. Prevalence of obesity, diabetes, and obesity-related health risk factors. *Journal of the American Medical Association* 289(1):76–79.

Narayan, K. M., J. P. Boyle, T. J. Thompson, S. W. Sorensen, and D. F. Williamson. 2003. Lifetime risk for diabetes mellitus in the United States. *Journal of the American Medical Association* 290(14):1884–1890.

National Fund for Medical Education. 2006. *Advancing community health worker practice and utilization: The focus on financing*. San Francisco: Center for the Health Professions, University of California at San Francisco.

National Standards for Culturally and Linguistically Appropriate Services in Health Care ([Final Report] U.S. Department of Health and Human Services, Office of Minority Health). 2001. http://www.omhrc.gov/assets/pdf/checked/finalreport.pdf (accessed April 10, 2007).

Norris, S. L., P. J. Nichols, and C. J. Caspersen. 2002. The effectiveness of disease and case management for people with diabetes. *American Journal of Preventive Medicine* 22:15–38.

Olsen, S. 2003. *Social return on investment: Standard guidelines*. Center for Responsible Business, 2003. http://repositories.cdlib.org/crb/wps/8 (accessed April 10, 2007).

PolicyLink. 2004. *The influence of community factors on health*. http://www.policylink.org/pdfs/AnnotatedBib.pdf (accessed April 4, 2008).

Robinson, R. G. 2005. Community development model for public health applications: Overview of a model to eliminate population disparities. *Health Promotion Practice* 6:338–346.

Rosenthal, E. L. 1998. *A summary of the National Community Health Advisor Study.* Annie E. Casey Foundation and the University of Arizona. http://www.rho.arizona.edu/Resources/Studies/cha-study/default.aspx (accessed April 11, 2008).

Sampson, R. J. 2003. Neighborhood-level context and health: Lessons from sociology. In *Neighborhoods and Health,* edited by I. Kawachi and L. F. Berkman. New York: Oxford University Press.

Sisk, J. E., P. L. Hebert, C. R. Horowitz, M. A. McLaughlin, J. J. Wang, and M. R. Chassin. 2006. Effects of nurse management on the quality of heart failure care in minority communities: A randomized trial. *Annals of Internal Medicine* 145:273–283.

Smith-Bindman, R., D. L. Miglioretti, N. Lurie, L. Abraham, R. B. Barbash, J. Strzelczyk, M. Dignan, W. E. Barlow, C. M. Beasley, and K. Kerlikowske. 2006. Does utilization of screening mammography explain racial and ethnic differences in breast cancer? *Annals of Internal Medicine* 144(8):541–553.

Wagner, E. H. 1998. Chronic disease management: What will it take to improve care for chronic illness? *Effective Clinical Practice* 1(1):2–4.

Weir, H. K., M. J. Thus, B. F. Hankey, L. A. Ries, H. L. Howe, P. A. Wingo, A. Jemal, E. Ward, R. N. Anderson, and B. K. Edwards. 2003. Annual report to the nation on the status of cancer, 1975–2000, featuring the uses of surveillance data for cancer prevention and control. *Journal of the National Cancer Institute* 95:1276–1299.

Williams, D. R., H. W. Neighbors, and J. S. Jackson. 2003. Racial/ethnic discrimination and health: Findings from community studies. *American Journal Public Health* 93:200–208.

Zerhouni, E. 2003. Medicine. The NIH roadmap. *Science* 302:63–72.